Beyond Chocolate

How to stop yo-yo dieting and lose weight for good

Sophie Boss and Audrey Boss

PIATKUS

✿ Visit the Piatkus website!

Piatkus publishes a wide range of best-selling fiction and non-fiction, including books on health, mind, body & spirit, sex, self-help, cookery, biography and the paranormal.

If you want to:

- read descriptions of our popular titles
- buy our books over the internet
- take advantage of our special offers
- enter our monthly competition
- learn more about your favourite Piatkus authors

VISIT OUR WEBSITE AT: www.piatkus.co.uk

First published in Great Britain in 2006 by
Piatkus Books Ltd
5 Windmill Street, London W1T 2JA
email: info@piatkus.co.uk

The moral right of the author has been asserted

A catalogue record for this book is available from the British Library

ISBN 0 7499 2708 9

Text design by Paul Saunders
Edited by Jan Cutler

This book has been printed on paper manufactured
with respect for the environment using wood from
managed sustainable resources

Typeset by Phoenix Photosetting, Chatham, Kent
Printed and bound in Great Britain by
MPG Books, Bodmin, Cornwall

For our two best role models: our mother, who showed us how far you can get when you are passionate about what you do . . . and how to throw *the best* party; and our father, a generous, kind leader who has backed us unreservedly all the way.

Contents

Acknowledgements   vii
Life Beyond Chocolate   1

1   The all-or-nothing trap   13

Tune in
2   Back to basics   28

Eat when you are hungry
3   Save that slice of cake for later, when
you're hungry   34
4   The answer to a problem is not always a
cup of tea and a biscuit . . . or ten   47

Eat whatever you want
5   Chocolate sandwiches for breakfast   64

Put it on a plate, sit down and focus
6   Eating crisps by candlelight   84

Stop when you are satisfied
7   Just how much is enough?   94
8   You are not a dustbin   106

Enjoy
9   Eating chocolate, without the guilty aftertaste   116

Own your body

10 Mirror, mirror on the wall   128
11 Every item in my wardrobe fits just right   144

Move!

12 Work it out   152

Support yourself

13 Asking for help, not a second helping   162

Be your own guru

14 Who's the expert?   174
15 The two-letter word   182
16 Making it happen   191
17 FAQs: Yes, but . . . what if?   199

Notes   206
Log on for more   209
The Chocolate Fairy's favourite resources   215
Beyond Chocolate workshops   223
Guru work   225
Further reading   241
Index   243

Acknowledgements

It's thanks to the vision and intuition of our agent David Riding at MBA that you are reading this book. His encouragement and support turned our initial hesitation into enthusiasm. His work in helping us shape this book has been invaluable and we will never forget the delight, excitement and joy we felt when we left his office after our first meeting. He has supported us all the way, with good humour, warmth and integrity. He is a gem of an agent!

Our editor Jo Brooks was open minded and interested from the start; coming on one of our workshops to really understand what Beyond Chocolate is all about. Her goodwill and helpful suggestions have been of enormous value to the exciting and sometimes challenging process of writing *Beyond Chocolate*! We are grateful to her and all at Piatkus who believed in this book from the very start.

Many thanks to Surinder Phull who checked over the more scientific bits and patiently explained and re-explained the finer points of nutrition.

Beyond Chocolate would simply not have been the same without our many loyal and valued participants who made such poignant and candid contributions. We are truly grateful for their generosity and the honesty with which they shared their stories and experiences.

Sophie: Ben, Jasper and Evie have been so understanding and supportive of my late nights and early mornings at the PC, weekends away and hours on the phone. I appreciate them enormously. Jasper and Evie are continuous sources of inspiration and my best teachers, and Ben's love continues to nourish me year after year.

I can't imagine writing this book without my experience at Spectrum. Everything I have learned among my colleagues on the One Year (and beyond) and from Judy Hargreaves's warmth and wisdom is woven into the fabric of this book and I am so glad that I made my way there.

I am grateful beyond words to the women in my life: to Foxy whom I love and trust like a sister, to Liz for always being interested and encouraging, to RA, Gale, Dawn, Becky and Sophie who have listened, supported, challenged and held me, month after month over the years. And to Karen, Kate M, Jac and Emma whose friendship I treasure. A huge thank you to Mary for empowering me to run like the wind!

I value my long conversations with Geoff and Pete about the business side of Beyond Chocolate. I have felt gently challenged and always supported.

And finally I am so grateful to Audrey. I could never have dreamed that we would be so close and such good friends and that working together and writing together could be just so perfect! I love the way we spark off each other and how we know exactly what the other is thinking. Over the months of writing she has been so patient when I have been at my most trying, and calm and level when I have sparked off in all directions. Most of all I love laughing with her until I cry and until my sides feel like they're about to burst!

Audrey: I am so grateful to the many fantastic women I have met whilst roaming the world and who have given me the precious gift of friendship. A special thank you to Claudia, Marjorie, Sabrina, Kim and Catherine for the cups of tea, the phone calls and the emails; for always being there to celebrate the good times and provide words of wisdom when everything goes pear shaped. You have, over the years, been a continuous source of inspiration, laughter and food for thought, much of which has found its way into these pages.

Johnny has looked on patiently while his flat was invaded by piles of books, bits of computer equipment and a lot of pink stuff. His belief in Beyond Chocolate, his thoughtfulness and the massive doses of TLC he lavishes upon me have repeatedly rekindled my sometimes waning enthusiasm in writing this book. Thank you for showing me how good it can be.

Sophie's passion and vision are the driving force behind Beyond Chocolate. I can't imagine writing this book with anybody else. She's the only person I know who can debate the word order of a sentence with a blender in one hand, her mobile in the other, pausing occasionally to admire a drawing and yet never lose the thread. The energy and dedication she puts into every aspect of her life are infectious and her compassion and integrity are inspirational. Thank you for being sister, best friend and mentor all rolled into one!

Life Beyond Chocolate

Can you imagine a life without the slavery of dieting and constantly controlling your weight? A life without rules about what and how much you eat, without having to 'be good'? Just imagine how it would feel to get up in the morning without having to face the dreaded scales; to get dressed and wear clothes you love and feel good in; to think of food only when you are hungry; to enjoy, savour and celebrate every meal; to eat your favourite foods without counting calories, calculating fat content or feeling guilty. And how liberating it would be to feel truly nourished and satisfied, whatever you've eaten; to find a way of moving your body that you enjoy, and that leaves you feeling alive and full of energy; to go out to a fabulous restaurant without having to settle for the 'healthy option'.

In a life Beyond Chocolate, you will have a relaxed, healthy relationship with food and your body. And the beauty of it is that along the way you'll shed the extra pounds and you'll never have to worry about putting them back on.

The Beyond Chocolate approach works because it takes us back to how our bodies are supposed to function. Everybody can do it, it's just that after years of listening to the experts, going on diets and following self-imposed weight-loss crusades, you've forgotten how to. All you need to do is discover how to listen to your body again. In this book we will show you how.

You may be wondering who 'we' are and how Beyond Chocolate came about. We are sisters, Audrey and Sophie.

Audrey I went on my first diet when I was 13. My mother stood me in front of the mirror in my underwear and asked me if I really wanted to go to the beach looking like *that*. I spent the next three months on the Mayo Clinic diet, mostly eating poached fish, hard-boiled eggs, tomatoes and apples. I lost weight, a lot of weight and, delighted by the results, started to cut down on the already meagre portions allowed by the programme. By the time the summer came round I was looking, to my eyes, pleasantly skinny – and fainting regularly from lack of food.

September rolled round, and it was back to boarding school. Buttered toast at breakfast, and tea and sweets from the village shop became my only form of sustenance as I refused to eat the revolting school meals on offer, and I rapidly regained all the weight I had lost – plus a little more. This was the beginning of a 20-year cycle in which I yo-yoed between losing weight and then putting it all back on again. I tried everything: diet books, doctors who prescribed hunger suppressants, WeightWatchers, home-made eating plans based on calorie counting, and countless other miracles that promised me a thin body. I even used vomiting as a way of controlling my weight.

It became harder and harder to stick to the diets, I 'slipped up' more and more frequently with longer and more intensive 'pig-out' periods. And I always seemed to put on more weight than I had lost. By the time I was in my mid twenties I was starting a new diet, or vowing to 'be good and watch what I ate' every Monday morning. These attempts lasted anything from until lunchtime to a few days, before I gave up and went off the rails – until the Monday after.

The more weight I put on, the more miserable I became, and the more miserable I was, the more I ate. I hated my body with a passion; hated my flabby stomach, which bulged out over the waist of the too-tight jeans I squeezed myself into; hated the rolls of fat on my back and the flaps under my arms, which I covered up with baggy T-shirts; hated my triple chin, which I couldn't hide. Against all logic I believed that my weight was at the root of all my problems and that if only I were thin, I would be happy.

My ongoing battle with obsessive dieting, bulimia and a destructive body image was very private. I never talked about it to anyone. Not to my girlfriends, who were all thinner than me, not to my boyfriend, who I knew would tell me to 'just get a grip and eat less', not to my sister, who was forever embarking on a new weight-loss crusade herself, and not to my mother, who had been consistently depriving herself for the past 40 years in a systematic cycle of starving during the week and bingeing on weekends.

Anyone looking at me from the outside would have seen an outgoing, friendly woman who was good at her job and had a lively social life. I never talked about the self-loathing, about the late-night binges, or about the vomiting. After all, I felt it was entirely my fault, that I was weak and pathetic, and simply lacked the willpower to go on a diet, lose weight and sort myself out once and for all. So I kept quiet and kept going round and round in circles.

I moved to Rome and set up a new life in Italy – and ate. I threw myself into my work, building up a successful freelance career in PR and event management – and ate. I travelled and I discovered new worlds – and ate. I went out and had fun – and ate. The years went by and I continued to pile on the pounds. By the time I was 30 I was overweight, desperately unhappy with my body, running out of options and ready for change.

This book is about how that change began. It came about first and foremost by accepting that the way I was approaching weight loss was not only completely ineffective but it was also harmful, not only to my health but also to my self-esteem and ultimately to my happiness. It came about by being willing to put lifelong beliefs into question, by being open to new, and sometimes daunting ideas, by experimenting and learning from my experiences. It came about, above all, thanks to my sister Sophie. She was the person I turned to when I finally decided to open up and talk about my struggle with food. That was when I discovered that we had been going through the same thing for years, without ever talking about it. It is thanks to her support and vision that I found the courage to make changes.

Since then, we have come a long way. My life as an unhappy, overweight, serial dieter has been transformed. All the energy, time and effort I used to put into trying unsuccessfully to lose weight in the past has been freed up and goes into more joyful, rewarding and enriching activities. Today, I have a life Beyond Chocolate.

Sophie Just like my sister, I spent most of my adult life from the age of about 13 to 34 either on a diet or eating for Britain. I remember very well the first time I dieted; it was at boarding school, with my best friend. We decided that we would have a bowl of All Bran with skimmed milk for breakfast followed by two Ryvitas with Marmite for lunch and the same for dinner! I lasted about two days. Over the years I went on every diet in the book and made up many more of my own. I believed with all my heart that if I could just lose weight and be *thin* then everything would fall into place. When I was thin, men would find me attractive. When I was thin, I would be worthy of my mother's love and acceptance. When I was thin, then I could start dressing and behaving like a real woman. But until then, I would continue to feel like a fat middle-aged blob. I went to nutritionists and naturopaths; I tried detoxes and meal replacements and I even earned myself the WeightWatchers' Gold Card. I was so desperate to lose weight that I would go hungry for days on end, trying to starve myself into thinness following some outrageous new fad. Sometimes I lost weight, but mostly I didn't, and I *always* put it back on. And every time this happened I felt like a total failure. And yet, I never gave up: I read diet books like novels, avidly absorbing every word, hoping with all my heart that they would work. And they rarely did. The only times I ever lost weight and kept it off for any length of time were when I fell in love or started an exciting new job. And as soon as the novelty wore off, I was back where I started, cramming in the packs of salami and cakes, wishing I wasn't so out of control.

By the time I was 34 I was living in my dream house in London, home educating the children, doing an MA in Education and even managing my husband's company accounts; I had good friends and was a confident and capable woman in so many areas of my life, but somehow I didn't really appreciate any of it. I hated my body: my breasts were too big, my bum too wide, my thighs too flabby. I felt huge and miserable, I thought about dieting and losing weight all the time. And I ate constantly.

One day sitting at Audrey's kitchen table in Rome it all came tumbling out. When Audrey told me how for years she had been struggling, just like I had, I couldn't believe it. We had grown up together and neither of us had ever said a word. That's when I decided to take action. I made it a priority; I knew that I did not want to spend the rest of my life on diets, feeling like a failure. Transforming my relationship with food, changing old beliefs, patterns and behaviours was a daunting prospect, but I stopped dieting and went on a mission. I read every book I could lay my hands on. I kept a journal where I wrote about all the ideas, tools and methods I was exploring and experimenting with, those that I had ditched and those that had worked for me.

My commitment wavered at times and I learned to be patient and to be kind to myself in the process. As I gradually started making changes I realised the one thing I needed more than anything else was support, but there was none around. That's when I decided to use my own experience, knowledge and skills as a starting point to create a programme that I could offer women to support them (and myself in the process) to stop yo-yo dieting, to stop food controlling my life. I knew that my body would reach its natural healthy weight if I focused on having a healthy relationship with food.

I spent the next 18 months researching, talking to women and writing, creating Beyond Chocolate and working on my own relationship with food and my body. The more I worked at it the easier it became, and I lost weight without it ever being my focus. Eating had finally become a pleasurable life-sustaining activity – no more, no less – and when I looked in the mirror and saw a slimmer body, that's all it was, a slimmer body. Still me. I wasn't the perfectly happy, sorted woman I'd dreamed of. I spent hours on the phone to Audrey talking about it all and we bounced ideas off each other. I turned to her for advice on marketing and PR, and her encouragement and enthusiasm spurred me on.

However, I encountered resistance when I offered Beyond Chocolate to health clubs and other organisations, due to my lack of 'qualifications'. So I began training as a Humanistic psychotherapist. My training informs the work I do in many positive ways and gives me valuable tools, which I incorporate into the structure of the workshops. What began as professional development has become as much about learning to become a person as it has about developing my professional skills.

When I was finally ready to run the first weekend workshop, I knew that Audrey had to be there.

That's when 'we' became 'Beyond Chocolate'.

We ran our first workshop as a pilot and were thrilled by the experience. We knew that Beyond Chocolate had worked for us, that it was a precious gem, but we had no idea just how mind-blowing the participants would find it.

As we sat in the drawing room of a gorgeous country home with women from every walk of life, of every age, and from the four corners of the UK, we were bowled over by the stories that came tumbling out. We had always known that we couldn't possibly be the only ones to have such destructive, obsessive relationships with food and, yet, hearing it first hand from complete strangers was a revelation to every woman in the room. There was a sense of solidarity and understanding – every woman there knew that she was no longer alone in her struggle. As the weekend unfolded we saw all the participants go through a process of wonder and understanding. There were many light-bulb moments as we outlined the basic Beyond Chocolate principles and gave the participants the tools to put them into practice.

The women left on the Sunday, empowered and moti vated with a radically new mindset. Reading their feedback forms brought tears to our eyes; it was moving to realise the impact that Beyond Chocolate would make to their lives. The icing on the cake was to discover that Audrey and I loved working together; we complemented each other perfectly and made a fantastic team. So we ran more and more workshops and, as we evolved, so did the workshops.

What started as a weekend workshop based on the ideas that we had brought together from different sources turned into a philosophy which is uniquely our own. The more we learned, the more it became Beyond Chocolate. We owe this learning to our personal experiences, to our continued commitment to growing and learning and to the hundreds of women who have taken part in our workshops. By drawing on our personal experiences and infusing it with our qualities we have turned Beyond Chocolate into a series of workshops that are completely different from anything else.

Our principles are not rocket science; everyone knows that if you eat just what your body needs and you *move* you will lose weight. We won't be telling you to go away and do it. Instead, we will show you exactly *how*. We know that if we gave you a detailed plan to follow you wouldn't stick to it for any longer than the last diet or lifestyle change you went on. Beyond Chocolate is unique because we give you the tools to find the right approach that works for you – one that you will do every day because *you* thought of it, *you* decided and it fits into *your* life.

Beyond Chocolate is based on ten simple principles that, when put into action, give us all a completely new attitude to eating. They are not guidelines or rules that are one-size-fits-all commandments telling us what we should do, and the idea is not about following them to the letter (like a diet). Fit them into your life in any way that works for you. They even work in isolation – apply any one of these and you will be making valuable and positive changes to your approach to weight loss.

Tune in

Eat when you are hungry

Eat whatever you want

Put it on a plate, sit down and focus

Stop when you are satisfied

Enjoy

Own your body

Move!

Support yourself

Be your own guru

If you eat when you are hungry and stop when you are satisfied, eat all the foods you want without depriving yourself and enjoy moving your body, you will lose weight. And the best way to make sure you stay motivated and focused is to find ways of supporting yourself along the way. This book explains these principles in detail and outlines a manageable and enjoyable approach to overcoming all the obstacles that stand in the way of integrating these principles into your life: comfort eating, cravings, overeating, social situations, body image and much more.

We know this approach works, not only from our own experience but also from the continuous stream of enthusiastic testimonials that workshop participants have sent us over the years. We have had so many different women on our workshops; most of them arrive desperately wanting to lose weight. Yet when they tell us how Beyond Chocolate has changed their lives, what they all talk about is how free they feel, how they love being able to eat everything without feeling guilty, how they enjoy food rather than being controlled by it and how fit, healthy and comfortable they feel in their bodies. The weight loss is usually the last thing mentioned. It has become the welcome by-product of a healthy relationship with food.

Pippa Kerslake, from London, did a weekend workshop in Dorset

❝ Beyond Chocolate has made a big difference to me and has greatly changed my relationship with food. It has given me the confidence to stop dieting and trust myself to make my own decisions about what I fancy eating and when, after years of always being told what and when to eat on a diet. Now I really enjoy eating everything without feeling guilty. I'm not a prisoner to food any more. I'm much happier and more confident about my body and I've lost two stone, which really shows me I'm doing the right thing for myself. **)**

What makes Beyond Chocolate so special is that it's not just a theory to us. We are not experts or specialists or doctors; we don't purport to know better, or attempt to blind you with science. Beyond Chocolate wasn't created by a marketing team in the headquarters of a dieting industry giant, nor is it the 'brain child' of an ex-actress or of some obscure American professor. We are just two ordinary women who have found an alternative that works and are passionate about empowering other women to do the same. Today we feel we have come far enough to write it all down. This book encapsulates everything we have learned over the years about how to stay off the diets and lose weight by having a healthy relationship with food and our bodies.

We have strived to make this book interesting and readable, because we have found that so many how-to books are dry, prescriptive and patronising. The stories that you will find at the beginning of each chapter, in the sections entitled Before, Now and What happened? are all 100 per cent fact. Everything we write about happened to one or both of us. These narratives faithfully retrace the steps that lead us to a life Beyond Chocolate. We chose to write them in the first person, merging experiences from both our lives, although in some ways we are reflecting the experiences of so many women. 'I' could be Audrey, 'I' could be Sophie – 'I' could be you. We wrote every single word of this book together. We brainstormed, debated and polished every sentence. The 'I' is truly a blend of us both.

The book is divided into sections for each Beyond

Chocolate principle and each chapter focuses on one of these principles. The Before and Now sections in each chapter describe our life before and beyond chocolate, whereas the What happened? section maps the transition between one and the next. We want to emphasise that nothing 'happened' as if by a miracle, we made changes by taking action, experimenting and being willing to make mistakes.

In the sections we have called Action! you will find the practical tools and strategies that you can put into practice to start making those changes *now*.

We haven't filled each chapter with endless worksheets and written exercises, because we found them distracting and never actually completed them when they appeared in other books. They got us thinking, but we never wrote anything down. In each chapter you will find some Food for thought questions. If you like writing, put pen to paper here. However, we also know that women who attend our workshops always find worksheets and other exercises useful so we have included some of them at the end of the book in the Guru work chapter. You can download these and much more from our website (www.beyondchocolate.co.uk) – we'll explain how in the Log on for more chapter.

Writing this book was an opportunity to verify our approach from a theoretical perspective, we already knew it worked in practice. We read up on a lot of research and we discovered that we could have found a study, a report or a statistic to prove just about anything. However, too much research is funded by people or organisations who have a vested interest in the outcome. We used our intuition and common sense in deciding what to believe, and we invite you to do the same. We have included the nuggets of information we found most fascinating and informative in the Reality check and Did you know? sections in each chapter.

On our workshops, we don't do all the talking; the

participants' contributions are a valuable and crucial part of the experience. We wanted to give them a voice in this book too. They speak in different ways. Some have actively contributed to the book by writing about a particular way in which their relationship with food and their body has changed, whereas many others have sent us emails, letters and testimonials, parts of which we have reproduced with their permission. You will also see that we have quoted things that participants have said on our workshops. We have changed their names to preserve anonymity; this is why they all have names starting with B.

Much as we all love precise timescales and measurable targets we cannot tell you how much weight you will lose or how long it will take. What we can tell you is that your relationship with food can start to change now. You have already taken the first step by picking up this book. How rapidly you start to feel the benefits depends on your pace and the extent to which you apply Beyond Chocolate to your life.

Revolutionising the way you approach weight loss and developing a new relationship with food is an exciting and liberating adventure in which every day is different. In Chapter 16, Making it happen, we describe the different stages you are likely to go through, and we outline how to put it all into action so that you can start living your life Beyond Chocolate now.

There is no right way to use this book. Dip in and out, read it from cover to cover, take action or mull it over. The important thing is to take it at your own pace and above all . . . ENJOY.

Beyond Chocolate is your passport to freedom.

CHAPTER • 1

The all-or-nothing trap

How easy is it to stick to a diet properly? Most of them are so restrictive and punishing that we will, sooner or later, put a foot wrong. By then we are so fed up that when we do break a rule we decide to break it properly and make the most of all those forbidden goodies that are off-limits in the diet before we get back on to the straight and narrow. You are either on the diet or off the diet. Following the rules to the letter or not doing it at all.

Before

Sunday evening, 8 pm I'm starting a new diet tomorrow. This one's going to work, they explain it really well, menu plans and all, so I can't go wrong this time. I'm going to do it properly. I'm ready. I've chucked out all the chocolate, biscuits, sweets and crisps. I've been to the supermarket and stocked up on salad, cottage cheese and low-fat yoghurts, chicken and healthy snacks and I've put a pack of chocolate digestives in the biscuit tin so that Johnny and the kids don't moan. Dreading Tim and Katie's get-together on Saturday though, he's such a good cook. I'll resist somehow. I've renewed my membership to the gym and from now on I'll be going three times a week – no excuses this time. Hoping to persuade Helen to do the step aerobics class with me instead of our usual Wednesday film night – we just end up pigging out on popcorn and Maltesers anyway. I feel really motivated, I've got to fit into my little black dress for the Christmas party! It will work – it has to.

Monday, 10 pm Exhausted. Aerobics fab. All going great! This one's a winner. Fingers crossed.

Tuesday, 5 pm Cristina from graphics just came round with a home-made coffee walnut cake. I'm so proud of myself, I wasn't even tempted. I felt a bit mean because she made it herself and looked a bit put out when I said I couldn't have any. Now they'll all be in the kitchen tucking in. Aarrghhhh!

Wednesday, 2 pm I've just come back from the gym. Feel fantastic. It's going really well. And I haven't even had time for lunch, which is great, it means I can double the portion sizes tonight!

Thursday, 11 am Really chuffed, weighed myself this morning and I've lost a pound already! Feel a bit peckish but I've just had my mid-morning snack, so I'll have to wait until lunchtime. Oatcakes aren't that bad when you get used to them. Oh, I know, I'll have a coffee.

Thursday, 5 pm Damn! Cristina came round with another bloody home-made cake today. I just had to have a slice. I don't believe I did that but this one looked amazing and even had that creamy icing on top I can never resist. OK, no harm done, it's just one slice. Going to the gym tomorrow anyway, I'll do another 20 minutes on the rower, that's bound to be at least 300 calories isn't it? I'll look it up in the book.

Friday, 10 am New day, new resolve. Back on track. Little black dress here I come!

Friday, 6 pm Helen just called, can't make the aerobics class tonight, I'm pretty tired anyway and it's pouring out there. Think I'll curl up and watch telly.

Friday, 11 pm Just ploughed my way through what was left of the choc digestives, I feel sick. Hope they don't notice. I'll get some more tomorrow.

Saturday, 6 pm Oh God, nothing fits, nothing to wear, I'll to have to go to Tim and Katie's in my fat jeans. I hate them!

Sunday, 10 am Shit, shit, shit!!!!!!!!! I'm such a failure, why can't I just stick to it? I've got no willpower. I can't believe it. It's all those delicious jams, chutneys and cheeses that Tim brings back from Portugal, I just have to taste them all and they are so bloody good – and that was before dinner. Stuffed my face all night and now Johnny's parents have invited us for tea. Might as well just ditch it for today, I've blown it anyway, so what's the point.

Sunday, 8 pm God Michele's cheesecake's good. Had two slices 'cause that's it till Christmas. Starting again tomorrow, properly this time. I know I can I do it. I just need to stop giving in all the time and keep thinking about my little black dress. I can't be the fattest woman at the Christmas party. I just can't!

Repeat cycle!

Now

Dieting is one of a long list of words that has been relegated to the dictionary dustbin along with lifestyle changes, healthy eating, being good, menu plans, calories, BMI, detox, and experts – I don't have rules any more. I am inspired by a set of principles that I constantly update, revise and evolve. I don't stick to these principles religiously, they define a general approach to eating and the way I feel about myself and my body. Every time I do something positive I'm taking a step in the right direction. I don't want to be perfect and I don't expect to get it right 100 per cent of the time. I know it's not possible to be perfect anyway. I don't yo-yo between all or nothing any more. If I want a piece of cake with my cup of tea even though I'm not hungry, that's fine. I eat it, and enjoy it. It doesn't mean that I have to pig out all day or make up for it by skipping lunch. I'd love to go swimming three times a week and when I manage one or two that's one or two more than none at all. There is no such thing as failure or success, only experiences to learn from.

What happened?

Deep down, I knew that dieting wasn't the answer, but I couldn't imagine doing anything else, and then one Monday morning as I tried to drag myself out of bed to go running in the park I felt a wave of despair wash over me. I had just started a high-protein lifestyle programme that was going to transform me. This was the miracle solution I had been looking for. I would lose weight, become fit and toned, and finally have the body I so desperately wanted. I hoped this one would work because it wasn't only a diet, it also included a daily exercise programme. I might actually stick to it because you got every seventh day off . . . on Sundays I got to pig out and eat anything I wanted! And it only lasted 12 weeks. Surely I could manage that? By then, I'd be ready for the beach.

Yet part of me already knew I wouldn't stick to it. Who was I kidding? I wasn't going to stick to this one for any longer than I'd stuck to all the others. Whether I kept it up for a few days or miraculously managed the whole 12 weeks, and even if I did lose weight, I knew that sooner or later I'd put it all back on and I'd be back to square one. As I lay there battling with these thoughts, the voice of despair got louder and suddenly it all felt like a long, hard, impossible slog. I knew it would only get worse with the sense of inevitable failure that awaited me a few days later as I gave in to some chocolate in front of the telly or missed my morning run because I couldn't drag myself out of my warm bed.

Why was it so difficult to lose weight? What was wrong with me? It couldn't be that hard to eat sensibly and shift some pounds. I felt so miserable and hopeless. I would never get out of this bottomless pit.

It was clear that dieting wasn't working. Every time I launched myself into another weight-loss crusade I ended up feeling like a total failure. For every pound I lost, I put one back on – plus a little more, and it was getting harder and harder to lose weight. By going on yet another diet, I knew that I would be back where I started before I could blink, yo-yoing miserably for the rest of my life.

The alternative, though, was to stop dieting and controlling what I ate; and that was unthinkable. All my life I had been controlling my weight because that's what women did. If you wanted to lose weight and be thin, you had to diet or at the very least control what you ate very carefully. If I wasn't doing that, how was I going to manage? I'd never stop eating and I'd end up as big as a house. If I didn't watch what I ate I'd be totally out of control and eating anything that wasn't tied down. But I had tried everything and the options were running out.

Thinking about it, my experience told me that being 'on' a diet was always followed by being 'off' the diet. Being good and depriving myself was always followed by overindulging and eating all those fattening, unhealthy foods that I didn't allow myself when I was on a diet. It stood to reason, then, that not being on a diet at all was bound to change something! If there was no 'on' then surely there could be no 'off'. I knew that yo-yo dieting was bad for my health as well as my self-esteem, so it was worth a try at the very least.

Being the Internet and Amazon enthusiast I am, I logged on to see if there was anything out there about this. There wasn't much, but to my delight I did find a few books and websites that advocated ditching the diets and approaching weight loss from a different angle. I ordered the books and trawled through the web pages. It was a revelation. What these women were saying was that it wasn't my fault if I couldn't stick to the diet; that I wasn't pathetic, weak-willed and a failure. It was the diets that had failed me because they didn't work – for anyone.

These books encouraged me to stop dieting and they provided some incredibly useful suggestions on how I could transform my relationship with food forever. I read and read and read. I wrote and kept a record of what I was going through and about how my relationship with food was changing. I went to see a therapist. I found an ally in my sister who was going through the same experience and we supported each other. I made small changes, one step at a time. Gradually, I learned to think and behave differently and I changed my approach to eating and to weight loss; not by reprogramming my mind or using any special techniques but simply by experimenting with different ideas and, above all, noticing what I experienced and learning from it. I knew that I was in the process of creating new habits. I didn't have to stick to this new approach religiously all the time, and even if a few days or weeks went by when I didn't, I could still come back to it over and over again. The more I did it, the more natural it became.

What it boils down to

All diets and their cousins are the same. They are based on a set of rules to be followed scrupulously. If you don't follow them, they won't work. Sometimes it's called 'healthy eating' or 'being good', sometimes it's touted as a lifestyle change. Recently diets have slipped in through the back door as a 'detox'. Whatever they are called, they all equate to the same thing: *any* programme or plan that tells you what or what not to eat, when to eat it and how much of it to eat is a diet. And diet mentality means being stuck in the all-or-nothing trap. You're either on it or off it. Doing it properly or not doing it at all.

Rules are meant to be broken

How many women do you know who are on a diet, in between diets or working hard at staying slim? The problem is: diets are impossible to follow. The diet mentality requires us to be perfect. No slip ups allowed. We tell ourselves that willpower is the key to sticking to the rules and reaping the rewards. But none of us has enough willpower to stick to a diet or maintenance plan forever. Few of us know how to, or even want to, deprive ourselves for a lifetime. Having rules can be reassuring. They give us a sense of control and the illusion that as long as we stick to them we are on the right track. Yet they are so counterproductive. After all, rules are meant to be broken. Impose a set of rules on yourself and the next thing you know you'll be finding ways to break them and you'll beat yourself up for not sticking to them properly.

Whether you last a week, a month or a year, eventually you'll give in. Deprivation and 'being good' are simply unsustainable in the long term. Diets trap us in an endless yo-yoing of success and failure, losing weight, then putting it all back on again.

The idea that diets don't work for long-term weight loss is nothing new. It's been studied, documented and proven beyond a shadow of a doubt. The figures speak for themselves: for every person who has lost weight and kept it off, there are nine others looking for the next magic wand. Many of the new weight-loss schemes are now claiming not to be diets when in fact they are just that. If they are giving us rules and guidelines to follow, if they include dos and don'ts they are diets. It's hard not to go on them, and there seems to be no alternative. Everywhere we look we are bombarded with promises of easy weight loss and miraculous transformations, by an industry that makes millions out of our unflagging hope.

Diets fail us because they address the problem the wrong way round

It's not losing weight we need to focus on, it's our relationship with food. Learning how to have a healthy, balanced, intuitive relationship with food leads to long-term weight loss, not focusing all our energy and efforts on getting rid of the weight, which is only the symptom. When we change our approach and learn to eat when we are hungry and stop when we are satisfied, as well as overcoming all the obstacles that stand in the way of doing that, weight loss becomes an inevitable by-product of that change. We can reach the weight that's right for us, without having to go on diets or depriving ourselves. The beauty of Beyond Chocolate is that since you are not 'on' a diet – or 'on' anything else for that matter – you won't be 'off' it, slip up, get it wrong or have to start again on Monday.

Billie, who was a veteran dieter, came on one of our weekend workshops having tried everything out there to lose weight. When we introduced the idea of ditching the diet mentality by stepping off the all-or-nothing treadmill, she was horrified and sceptical, 'How am I going to know if I'm doing it right if there are no rules to follow?'

This is how many participants react to this idea at the beginning when we explain that Beyond Chocolate is not about following a set of rules and prescriptions. What Beyond Chocolate does provide is an array of practical tools and strategies along with an understanding of our relationship with food.

That initial horror is long gone by the end of the workshop.

❛ It was brilliant on the weekend; I did not feel patronised in any way. I know everything there is to know about diets and nutrition and was so relieved to find that this is not what I was going to learn. ❜

Lexi Stavely-Hill

❛ Beyond Chocolate has given me the directions to get to a place I've always wanted to be at . . . I know I can become the me I've not even dared to dream of. THANK YOU! ❜

Jayne Hall

❝ I found this to be a truly powerful course . . . I take home lots of skills and new ideas to change my relationship with food. I think this will change my life. THANK YOU SO MUCH! ❞

Pippa Kerslake

❝ The principles of Beyond Chocolate are a revelation to me. The more I think about them, the more they make sense. I am leaving with a completely different mindset. ❞

Manuela Alcock Palazotta

❝ Excellent materials provided, I felt really special to be on a Beyond Chocolate workshop. After a truly wonderful weekend with like-minded women, I no longer have to start tomorrow any more. My life can start now. Good bye "on-and-off" mentality; hello "being free". ❞

Julie Jones

ACTION!

A good place to start:

How many diets have you tried out, and what expert advice have you followed over the years?

Below are all the ones that come up again and again on our workshops. We've done many of them ourselves; feel free to add your own.

The diets I have tried are:

Atkins	Low Carb
Ayurvedic	Low Fat
Beverly Hills	Magazine and book diets
Blood type	Making up my own diets
Cabbage soup	Mayo Clinic Diet
Carbohydrate Addicts	Metabolic Type Diet
Crash diets	OMEGA Diet
Detox (in general)	Pritikin Principle
Dieting during the week	Raw Food Diet
Dr Phil	Rosemary Connolly
Eat More, Weigh Less	Scarsdale Diet
Fit for Life	Scottish Slimmers
Food Combining	Slimfast
F-Plan Detox	Slimming Magazine Club
Glycaemic Index (GI) Diet	Slimming World
Glycaemic Load (GL) Diet	South Beach Diet
Gillian McKeith	Special K Challenge
Grapefruit diet	Sugar Busters
Herbal Integrators	The Cambridge Diet
Herbalife	The EGG Diet
High protein	Very low-calorie diet
Hollywood Diet	WeightWatchers
Lighter Life	Zone

Other ways I have attempted to control my weight:

Acupuncture	Consulting your GP
Adopting lifestyle changes	Eating smaller portions
Avoiding puddings	Eliminating food groups
Being 'good'	Exercising
Calorie counting	Fasting
Consulting nutritionists	Hypnosis

Seeing weight loss experts Using laxatives/diuretics
Surgery Using meal replacements
Taking hunger suppressants Vomiting
Therapy/counselling

Take stock of the diets you have been on and all the different ways in which you have attempted to control your weight. What kind of dieter are you? Can you see a pattern?

- Do you prefer dieting or do you find other ways of controlling your weight? Or maybe you have given up altogether?

- Do you like to follow the latest diet to the letter or do you prefer making up your own?

- Do you manage really well for a while and then give up, or do you sabotage yourself from day one?

- Do you do them, lose weight and then put it back on or do you just give up halfway through?

- Do you do them alone or prefer doing them with friends?

- Do you make them official and tell everyone, or do you do them in secret hoping no one will notice?

How many years have you spent dieting or wanting to lose weight? Take a moment to add up the years and look back at the list above. Since you are reading this book, it's more than likely that not one of these has given you what you want: permanent sustainable weight loss and a healthy relationship with food and your body.

Just think how liberating it is to know that you will *never* have to do any of these again. Ever.

REALITY CHECK

A study on the diet mentality

A study[1] by psychologists in Canada looked at the effect of food restrictions on willpower. The researchers found this quite difficult to study, because people change the way they act when they think they are being observed. So, they adopted a 'deceptive' methodology. Dieters and non-dieters were told that they were participating in a taste-preference study. They were given a variety of low- and high-calorie foods to 'sample' and comment on. They were thanked for their help in the study with a complementary buffet lunch. This is when the real research began. Unbeknown to the participants, research staff observed them behind two-way mirrors recording what and how much each participant was eating.

What they found was fascinating but not surprising. The dieters who had sampled low-calorie foods ate less than the non-dieters. They were on a diet after all. However, when the sample food used in the 'study' was high in calories, dieters consumed significantly more during the buffet than those who were not dieting! They had broken the diet for that day anyway, so there was no point in depriving themselves. After succumbing to one chocolate biscuit, it's easy to feel like a failure and adopt the all-or-nothing 'I've blown it today, I'll start again properly tomorrow' attitude . . . and finish off the whole packet. The idea that there would be a restriction in the future paradoxically motivated them to go against the restriction 'to get it while they could'.

? DID YOU KNOW . . .

- Fewer than 1 per cent of people who follow commercial diet programmes are able to maintain their weight loss for five years.

- Only 25 per cent of people are able to follow a diet plan closely for one year.

- The dieting industry banks on repeated failure and false hopes. After all, it would be a very short-lived business if dieters succeeded the first time.

I taste the freedom when . . .
I can't remember the last
time I even considered
dieting.

Food for thought

How many years have you spent dieting or trying to lose weight?

How do you feel about not having rules, guidelines or a set programme to follow?

How often you do fall into the all-or-nothing trap?

Tune in

Eat when you are hungry

Eat whatever you want

Put it on a plate, sit down and focus

Stop when you are satisfied

Enjoy

Own your body

Move!

Support yourself

Be your own guru

CHAPTER 2

Back to basics

Tuning in is like a golden thread that ties all the Beyond Chocolate principles together and you will find it woven in to many chapters of this book. It is about turning to yourself for the answers, listening to your body rather than looking to the 'experts'. Tuning in is nothing other than going back to basics and gathering information about how you feel physically, how you feel emotionally and what thoughts are going through your head at any given moment. The more information you have about yourself the easier it is to make changes in your approach to weight loss.

When you listen to your body you will begin to recognise the cues that let you know when you need food, what you want to eat and when it's time to stop. By tuning in you can break the hand-to-mouth action that often leads to an empty plate without you even noticing. You can eat just what your body needs and lose weight. You will find out what exercise you really love, how to motivate yourself to feel good and how to ask for help when you need it.

In each chapter we will be showing you exactly how to

tune in – it's straightforward and quick, and you won't need any special techniques, charts, gadgets or counters.

Eat when you are hungry

When you tune in and listen to your body you will recognise all your hunger cues, from the obvious, unmissable ones to the more subtle signals.

Eat whatever you want

Your body knows exactly what you need, and tuning in is the best way to find out. You will have a healthy balanced diet without depriving yourself of anything.

Put it on a plate, sit down and focus

It's so much easier to tune in when you are not rushing and eating on the go.

Stop when you are satisfied

When you tune into your body's signals you will know exactly how much is enough.

Enjoy

Food can be a delicious, nurturing, sensual experience. Why deprive ourselves of this pleasure! When you tune in it's so much easier to enjoy it.

Own your body

Tuning in can turn 'fat' days into a positive approach to body image.

Move!

Let your body tell you how it likes to move. Rather than sticking to an exercise regime, tune in and find out what you really enjoy.

Support yourself

Find out how to give yourself a helping hand – you're the one who knows what you need.

Be your own guru

Tuning in means looking to yourself for the answers and knowing that you are your own best expert.

Sarah Layton, from London, came on a weekend workshop in London

Before

❝ I didn't recognise what I was feeling – that I was tired, cold, sad or hungry, for example. I would feel "out of sorts", unable to concentrate, and would reach for chocolate or other food I considered "bad" and feel guilty. The eating would distract me from the moment of really strong feelings and enable me to go back to work – but it was a temporary relief.

When I couldn't hold the discomfort at bay with food I felt guilty because I felt that I should be able to discipline myself better when there was work to be done. I didn't look after myself well and felt that I was "not good enough, lazy, inefficient and disorganised". I thought that if I tried harder, planned ahead more and made more effort I could conquer what was wrong with me. ❞

Now

❝ I am more aware of myself and listen to myself sympathetically when I feel uncomfortable. I take notice when I am tired, cold, hungry or sad and I take my feelings seriously. I rest if I need to – sometimes just for 20 minutes – and it makes a huge difference to how I feel. I plan my meals for enjoyment not just for nourishment and sit down with a candle at the table to eat.

The upshot of these changes is that I am beginning to use food much less for comforting myself and dealing with difficult feelings and instead keep it just for when I am hungry. I am more able to feel my feelings – both physical and emotional – and so can often respond to them in a more useful and appropriate manner – by resting when I am tired, crying when I am sad and dressing more warmly when it is cold. I am generally kinder to myself and I like myself more. ❞

Tune in

Eat when you are hungry

Eat whatever you want

Put it on a plate, sit down and focus

Stop when you are satisfied

Enjoy

Own your body

Move!

Support yourself

Be your own guru

CHAPTER 3

Save that slice of cake for later, when you're hungry

Eating when you are hungry is the starting point for a healthy relationship with food, which in turn leads to weight loss. But how do you know when you are hungry? This may seem like an obvious question but the reality is that we are so out of touch with our bodies that many of us no longer know how to read the cues. Learning how to recognise and respond to these cues is a fundamental part of Beyond Chocolate.

Before

I knew how it felt to be ravenous or stuffed to bursting, but anything in between was a mystery. I ate when the clock told me to, on my lunch break, at family meal times. I ate when it fitted in with people's expectations. For years, hungry or not, I ate according to the rules of the latest diet I was following. I never once asked myself when it would suit *me* best to eat. It never even occurred to me that it might be an option. Most days I ate so often that I never felt hungry anyway. I ate breakfast and several mid-morning snacks before lunch. My afternoon cups of tea were the perfect excuse to dip into the biscuit tin. I picked while I cooked dinner and afterwards I nibbled the evening away – not hungry, just bored.

At the other extreme there were days when I managed to eat virtually nothing. I would get to that very hungry stage and go right beyond it; sometimes I would make it all the way to bed. More often, by early evening I would be ravenous and eat until I felt sick or needed to lie down. If I was offered a slice of cake at work, I found it almost impossible to say no. If I had already broken the diet, then what the hell! If I had been 'good' then I might be able to resist, but mostly not. And eating that slice of cake certainly had nothing to do with how hungry I felt. I was fighting a constant battle between eating as little as possible and my desperate desire to eat anything that wasn't tied down.

Now

I eat when I am hungry. When I tune in my body tells me very clearly just how hungry I am, the cues are crystal clear and I know what they mean. I don't need to remind myself to tune in any more, it has become second nature. I recognise the cues in the same way that I know I need a wee or a drink of water. It feels normal and uncontrived, and I barely think about it.

Eating when I'm hungry means that some days I eat more, some days I eat less. And I have learned how to manage my hunger so that if I'm planning a meal out and I *want* to be hungry I can make sure that I will be. I feel comfortable eating at times which may seem unorthodox or not eating when I'm expected to. In fact, just today I was invited to lunch at my mother's. It was a 'posh' affair with my extended family and other guests. Having had a big breakfast I was barely hungry when it was time to eat. For first course my mother had made one of my favourites: a delicious pasta dish of cherry tomatoes roasted with Parmesan, breadcrumbs and olive oil and . . . well anyway, I didn't have any, but asked if she would save my portion for later. I had a couple of bites of the main course (delicious fried calamari) and half a glass of white wine. Later on that evening, when I felt that familiar hungry feeling, I cycled over to her house and, while she was busy playing bridge on the terrace with her friends, I let myself into the kitchen and sat down to a plate of spaghetti. All the more mouth-watering for my hearty appetite!

What happened?

When I first came across the concept of eating when I was hungry I was not impressed. I told myself that since I wasn't hungry very often I would never get to eat. Then on reflection I realised that I did know what it was like to deprive myself all day and get home from work starving; when I was that hungry I didn't care what I ate and I usually ate far too much. So, I concluded, eating when I was hungry would either mean eating like a bird or stuffing my face. Neither sounded terribly appealing, or helpful for that matter. I was also worried about what people would think if I didn't eat when they did or if I pulled out my lunch at an 'odd' time. For some reason I automatically imagined that I would be hungry at awkward times.

Quite apart from the practical challenge, I knew deep down that if I ate only when I was hungry that would mean finding other ways to handle the times when I ate for comfort. That's when I realised that I actually didn't have a clue when I was hungry. And the only way to find out was to go back to basics and tune into my body. I did this by asking myself if I was hungry whenever I wanted to eat, and tuning into any physical sensations, thoughts or feelings connected to hunger. I started to notice all kinds of physical sensations, from the obvious rumbling tummy to a burning in my solar plexus (I didn't even know I had one of those until I started describing these feelings in detail and needed a word for that part of my body – it's just below the breastbone).

I noticed how, when I was ravenous, I couldn't think straight, I became murderous and panicky, and my stomach felt cavernous and empty. I realised that there was a point at which I was perfectly satisfied. At that stage I could feel a comfortable fullness in my belly, but there was room for more. I could leave food on the plate without feeling hungry. Emotionally, I wasn't feeling anything very strongly – just OK. The temptation to finish the food on my plate at that stage had nothing to do with hunger and was more about liking the taste or just not knowing how to stop.

I wanted my hunger to be predictable and convenient. Sometimes it was, but on other days it wasn't. Quite often I still ate when I wasn't hungry, but just noticing that and acknowledging it was a step in the right direction. And, very gradually, I began to make changes. Eating when I wasn't hungry started to become less and less satisfying. I became very familiar with the physical sensations that signal a need to eat, or the moment to stop. I recognised my emotional responses much more quickly. When I caught myself thinking about food or found my mind wandering away from the taste of my lunch to my next activity, I knew that I was nearing satisfaction. I was starting to find the whole process of discovery quite fascinating and exciting. As I looked back I realised that without forcing myself or making it into a rule, I was eating out of hunger more often than not and it was becoming more natural and easy to do.

What it boils down to

It sounds simple enough to eat when we are hungry, yet so many of us don't. We eat to satisfy all kinds of hungers and in response to a variety of external cues. Dieting has contributed to this by suggesting that someone else can tell us when it's the right time to eat. And yet hunger is such a basic, instinctive need. Babies cry for food when they need it. They feel the cues loud and clear and they make sure that we do too! Many babies who are not fed on demand soon learn not to trust themselves and their bodies but to rely on someone else deciding for them. As adults we've been taught to ignore our hunger cues in favour of following a timetable or plan that is not connected to our bodies. When we yo-yo diet or reduce our food intake we replace automatic internal regulators of hunger for conscious mental ones. What we are doing is teaching ourselves how to stop responding to our hunger cues.

Eating when it suits US

Not only have we lost the ability to recognise hunger cues but we also tell ourselves that somebody else knows best. We eat because the clock says it's lunchtime, because the experts say breakfast is the most important meal of the day, because we have been invited out to dinner and it's rude not to, because the diet plan we are following says that we should have an oatcake, half a pot of low-fat cottage cheese and an apple for our mid-afternoon break. It rarely occurs to us to question this, to ask ourselves 'Am I hungry?' This is a life-changing habit.

A couple of months ago I received an email from Beverly who was halfway through our 12-week multimedia course; she wrote:

6 I've been having an amazing time recently; it's all started to fall into place, without so much conscious effort. Once I tune in I can really hear my stomach telling me when to eat and when to stop. It's amazing because I never really listened before. I am definitely eating less, so I know I was eating far too much. And my habitual times of being "starving", such as after school time and when I finish work are not the times when I am actually hungry at all. So those were comfort-eating moments! Probably boredom. I'm really starting to feel in control and better about myself. 9

Beverly is the perfect example of someone who has made profound changes in her life by asking herself 'Am I hungry?' and regularly tuning in.

There is always a way

On our workshops participants bring up countless obstacles that stand in the way of them eating when they're hungry. What we hear in our support sessions is how, by experimenting and being creative, they have managed to find ways of overcoming them. Every problem has a solution.

On our last one-day workshop, Beatrice was worried that she wouldn't be able to eat at the office outside the usual lunch hour. Nobody else does. When we suggested she could take some food to work with her so that she could eat when she was hungry she thought that could be a solution but was still concerned about what people would think if they saw her eating at her desk. She played around with lots of possibilities and finally decided that it would work best if she used an empty meeting room where she could close the door, sit down and eat in peace for a few minutes if she needed to.

Recognising our hunger is a starting point, because once

we tune in and start listening to the cues our body sends out about hunger, we will also notice the cues that tell us what kind of food we are hungry for and when we have had enough. And that's what a balanced healthy relationship with food can look like: eating when we are hungry, eating what we want, and stopping when we are satisfied. Trust that your body will tell you when it's time to eat.

Kiri Harris, from Devon, came on a residential weekend in Gloucestershire

Before

❛ Of course I ate when I was hungry! I was just always hungry. That was a true statement. I simply hadn't acknowledged what I was hungry for. I still haven't a lot of the time but I do now know the difference between tummy hunger and something else hunger.

I hadn't realised how much I was relying on food for support. In fact I'd seemingly lost the ability to feel true hunger as I was eating every time I either felt tired or upset, bored, angry, fed up, frustrated or even when I was really happy or felt that I should congratulate myself. In fact, more or less at any time. ❜

Now

❛ I now realise that true hunger for food is very clear. It's a physiological state that your brain picks up on loud and clear; as clear as "I'm bursting for a wee!". Recognising this has allowed me to try to deal with other types of emotional hunger in different ways. I do still turn to the chocolate when I'm upset. I'm working on that, but there are now occasions, especially if I know I'm having a meal that I'm particularly looking forward to, that I allow myself to get properly hungry, not famished, but really ready to enjoy my meal and WOW! It tastes SO much better. And THAT'S what they mean when they say satisfied. I could never stop when I was satisfied because I was never really hungry in the first place! ⟩

ACTION!

A good place to start:

Tune in.
Begin by building up a picture of what your hunger feels like. Do this by tuning into your body. Do it now!

1. Tune into any physical sensations: what is your body telling you about your need for food? Is there a particular part of your body that is sending out strong cues? We all feel our hunger physically in different ways.

2. Notice any emotions connected to hunger. Do you feel any different emotionally when you are hungry, very hungry or starving?

3. What do you think about when you are hungry? Do you often think about the same things or find your mind wandering in the same way whenever you need food? When you are in a diet mentality you might think it's good to be hungry, that it means you will lose weight, and you ignore it as best you can. With Beyond Chocolate, feeling hungry means you eat.

With a little practice not only will you be able to tell exactly when you are hungry and when you are not but you will also recognise all the subtle levels in between. As you get more information, build up a picture of all the these levels when you tune in, from starving to stuffed, as well as the cues that you notice for each one.

On our workshops we use a scale from 0 to 5 where 0 equals ravenous and 5 equals stuffed. Use the scale below to describe the physical sensations, thoughts and feelings connected to each level so that you build a picture of how you get from 0 to 5. Every scale looks different because everyone's hunger is different. Create your own scale and update it regularly.

0   1   2   3   4   5

Example: 0 = ravenous

Physical I feel light-headed and nauseous. I am aware of feeling a burning sensation in my belly.

Emotions I am edgy, irritable and anxious.

Thoughts I can't focus on anything because I keep thinking about food.

Make it a habit

Next time you want to eat, spend *one* minute (that's all it takes) to tune in and find out how hungry you are. Do this several times a day, the more you practise the more natural it becomes. Eventually you will barely have to think about it.

Remembering to tune in can be a challenge, most of us are so used to *not* noticing ourselves that it takes practice. So make it as easy as possible: create reminders. Here are a few suggestions:

- Use the reminder on your mobile phone – you can set it to play a particular tune every time you want to remember to tune in.

- Use your PC alarm to do the same thing.

- Have a message on your screensaver. This could be an obvious one like 'Remember to tune in!' or it could be anything that would serve to jog your memory: Beyond Chocolate, for example!

- Stick Post-it notes around the place. You can write something on them or draw a smiley face, anything that will remind you of the reason you stuck them there in the first place. Stick them on your fridge, your bathroom mirror, in your diary, inside your travel card holder, inside your front door or on the dashboard of your car.

- Take one minute to tune in (that's all you need): when you sit down to a meal, when you wake up in the morning or before you go to sleep at night.

Start at the beginning

Wake up in the morning and instead of having your breakfast at the usual time, wait until you are hungry. How long does this take? How do you know when your body needs food? Tune in throughout the day. How long does it take you to get hungry again once you have eaten? Does it vary according to what and how much you have eaten?

When you are hungry – eat. And if you're not hungry and you eat anyway, don't beat yourself up. Tell yourself you are doing your best and focus on congratulating yourself when you do. Eat when you are hungry as often as you can and notice any patterns or triggers that lead you to eating when you're not.

Don't wait too long

If you wait until you're ravenous before you eat you are not likely to be very choosy about what you have – anything will do as long as it's NOW. It's easy to gobble food down fast when you are very hungry, and that's one of the surest ways to end up overeating. So aim to eat before you are famished.

Think ahead . . .

You might think that you will be hungry at times when it isn't convenient to eat or that food might not be to hand, so plan ahead. One way is to make sure that you have something with you. It's also worth remembering that a tea break or lunchtime is usually around the corner. Our lives tend to be structured in such a way that we can eat regularly. If yours is not, and you work from home or are on the go, for example, you can make a point of stopping what you are doing at regular intervals to eat if you are hungry. If you are not in a position to make decisions about break times or your work doesn't allow for regular breaks, you can ask for them. We all have the right to have regular breaks – wherever we are, whatever we are doing.

Going out

If you have been invited out to dinner and you're not hungry you could join your friends at the restaurant and just enjoy their company – a little unorthodox, but why not? It's better than settling for the dreary 'healthy salad' that you're not hungry for anyway.

REALITY CHECK

What happens to your body when you don't eat

Hunger is a signal from the body that it needs fuel. When you don't respond to these signals, whether through dieting or waiting for 'appropriate' times to eat, your body responds by going into starvation, or famine mode, as it is known in medical jargon.

By denying your body food when it needs it, you are telling it that there is none available – that you are starving – and it responds with a series of measures aimed at dealing with the emergency.

The first thing it does is to shut down and lower your metabolic rate in order to conserve energy. At the same time it becomes even more efficient at storing fat while waiting for new food supplies to replenish energy levels.

The body then sets about solving the crisis by sending out increasingly strong requests for fats and sugar: the best sources of instant energy. If starvation mode persists, the body will continue to activate emergency strategies and to start breaking down its own muscle tissue to convert into glucose (energy), leaving the fat stores intact, because it never knows when they might be needed.

When you do finally respond to your hunger – because, let's face it, nobody can go without food for very long – the extra fuel is stored as fat.

The longer and more frequently the body is in starvation mode, the better it gets at storing fat, as it never knows when fuel will next be available.

> ### ❓ DID YOU KNOW . . .
>
> Undernourishment affects people's health, productivity, sense of hope and overall well-being. A lack of food can stunt growth, slow thinking, sap energy, hinder foetal development and contribute to brain damage[1].

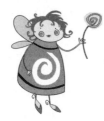

I taste the freedom when . . . I don't eat by the clock.

Food for thought

- ◉ If I ate only when I was hungry, I would . . .
- ◉ If I ate only when I was hungry, other people would . . .
- ◉ Are there any obstacles that stand in your way of eating when you are hungry?
- ◉ How will you get around them?

CHAPTER • 4

The answer to a problem is not always a cup of tea and a biscuit . . . or ten

If we eat when we are hungry, what do we do about all those times we want to eat when we are not hungry? By tuning in to the thoughts and feelings that are driving us to eat, instead of automatically reaching out for food, we can find other ways of truly nourishing ourselves.

Before

I spent so much time eating. I would get to work and head straight for the canteen for a hash brown and a sausage sandwich, having already had cereal and a cup of tea before I left home. That double breakfast provided the perfect distraction from my stressful job. I could legitimately kill half an hour in the canteen before heading up to my desk – after all, I was entitled to breakfast.

At lunch, hungry or not (and generally not) I would be really good and opt for the low-fat, healthy option and then spend all afternoon making endless cups of tea and regular trips to the vending machine. I would get home from work and make a beeline for the fridge, without even thinking. I'd open it and stare until I found something that beckoned, and that would be just the beginning.

Dinner just never seemed satisfying enough and I would spend the evening making repeated trips to the kitchen to eat a bit of this or a bite of that: a handful of cashew nuts, a few dried dates, cereal straight from the packet, a yoghurt with honey, a glass of fruit juice, a slice of cheese, pickles out of the jar with my fingers, more cashew nuts . . . until I felt nauseous and revolted at myself and at what I had eaten. Watching television wasn't the same without a big bowl of chocolate-covered peanuts or a pack of salami.

Sometimes I was exhausted at the end of the day, but for some reason I didn't want to go to sleep. I would take a book to bed with a bowl of something to nibble, anything really. Ideally crisps or nuts or salty snacks, but more often than not I didn't keep those foods in the house in a vain attempt to stop eating them, and so I would make do with Ryvita or matzo bread spread with butter and Marmite (fiddly but well worth it). I ate and read, with regular trips back for more, propping my eyes open until I fell asleep in the crumbs, full and disgusted.

I started these late-night excursions for food when I was about 13. I would creep out of my bedroom when everyone was asleep and tiptoe to the sitting room where the drinks cabinet was. Next to the whisky was a beautiful crystal bowl with a lid, which my mother always kept topped up with salted peanuts. I'd gently lift the lid and fill my little ramekin-sized bowl, replacing it carefully so as not to make that delicate pinging noise of crystal against crystal, lest any-one be alerted to my secret. Recently I discovered that my sister did exactly the same – it's a miracle we never bumped into each other!

Years later, when I was at home with children, I'd graze all day long as I tidied the house, took them to Tumbletots and wondered what I could do with the 20 minutes I had to myself while the baby had a nap. Bored and lonely at home alone, I would wander around and mysteriously find myself in the kitchen, yet again, opening cupboards and searching longingly, looking for something, anything.

Whether I was grazing my way through the day or having a major pig out, I always felt guilty and ashamed and would hate myself for my lack of willpower and self-control. It wasn't just at home or at the office, being on the move always involved eating. I went to the supermarket and bought a box of M&S lemon-drizzle slices as a treat. I told myself I would have just one straight away in the car park, but before I knew it they were nearly all gone and I stuffed in the last two because I couldn't take the evidence home with me.

A trip on the plane would mean filling up a rucksack with enough food to sustain me through a ten-day trek in the wilderness. On my way to Australia I consumed: three packets of Haribo liquorice wheels, a couple of large tubs of Pringles, three cartons of Ribena, two tuna sandwiches, a duck wrap, a tray of sushi, a family-sized pack of all-butter English toffees, an apple and two bananas, raisins, honey-roasted cashew nuts and a giant bar of Toblerone. Eating was a way of taking my mind off the fact that I was sitting in a tin can, miles above open water.

At dinners with family or friends I ate almost as if on automatic pilot. I didn't really taste the food, I just ate and ate and ate, until I couldn't fit in another crumb. These occasions were always a good excuse to eat because everyone else was doing it and I love good food. I filled myself up with food when in fact I wanted a fuller life, not a fuller stomach, only I didn't quite know how to swap one for the other.

Now

I eat when I'm hungry. I like it. I like feeling hungry and then satisfying my hunger with food. And there are times when frustration or loneliness or fatigue still lead me to the chocolate in the cupboard. I make a choice. Most of the time, I choose to acknowledge what I am feeling and allow myself to go ahead and feel whatever is bothering me. I know it will pass. And I know where to get support if I need it. On the odd occasion, I prefer the soothing, warming feeling of chocolate melting on my tongue. I enjoy the sensations with the full knowledge that I am not hungry, that I am using food to help me cope, to look after myself. I don't feel guilty, nor do I spiral into a frenzy of self-hatred and disgust. I acknowledge what I am doing; I put the food on a plate, I eat it, experience it, and then I move on. I know that sometimes using food as a plaster is easier than facing the *real* problem, whatever that may be. And when I don't stuff my feelings, fears and anxieties down with yet another slice of cake, I'm faced with dealing with what's really going on. I don't want to live my life numb. Even if it is not always easy, I would rather feel it than zone out. I am more alive, more empowered and more whole. Food will always be my Achilles heel, but now I am in control. My relationship with food is healthy and balanced, and as a result I maintain a steady weight that is healthy for me and feels good.

What happened?

I started to wonder why it was that I felt so out of control and miserable around food. I didn't see myself as having a 'problem', I didn't feel depressed and I wasn't overwhelmed or anxious. I was a happy and outgoing person who knew how to have fun. How I could I be so confident and 'together' in most areas of my life yet, somehow, lose the plot when it came to food?

I decided to start observing myself with the same fascination I had for those cookery programmes on television. I noticed when and how I ate when I wasn't hungry, whether it was dipping repeatedly into the biscuit tin with my cup of tea or ordering pudding at the end of a large meal at my favourite restaurant. I discovered that I binged (or grazed or indulged or treated myself) when I was in between diets or busy failing at one. The more I told myself I shouldn't, the more I seemed to eat.

I saw that eating helped to distract me from thinking about how bored I was or that I didn't want to go to work the next day or of that row I'd had on the phone with my mum. When I was eating, the creamy lusciousness of the fudge or the salty crunchiness of the crisps somehow blocked out strong emotions.

Once the bigger picture became clear, I began to notice the subtleties. As I observed myself closely, I became very aware of what I was doing. It wasn't only when I was sad, pissed off, or anxious. Eating also meant I could put things off, keep myself going at the computer for hours without wasting precious time for a lunch break, treat myself to something nice without having to ask anyone for anything.

The solution seemed simple enough: just stop doing it. I knew that I wanted to but I hadn't worked out what I could do instead. All the books I had read said: have a bubble bath, phone a friend, go for a walk. But if I had known how to do anything other than eat, I would have been doing those things in the first place. The idea of just stopping outright was too overwhelming. If the food was there, I had to have it. I couldn't just sit there and do nothing.

So, that's when I decided to experiment, not to see if I could stop myself, but to see if I could pause. For just one minute. Whereas stopping altogether seemed an impossible task, knowing that it was only for 60 seconds made it bearable. That precious minute gave me enough time to tune in. If I wasn't hungry, what was going on? Instead of just reaching for the food and cramming it in mindlessly that brief investigation could provide me with important information. I started to do this regularly, every time I reached for food and realised I wasn't hungry. I didn't always manage it. Sometimes I was rebellious, I didn't want to pause and tune in, I couldn't be bothered to stop for even a second, I wanted food and I wanted it NOW. Sometimes I completely forgot and only remembered about pausing after I had polished off the food and was sitting there feeling miserable.

When I did manage, sometimes nothing came up at all; all I could feel was a compelling need to eat. At other times, it was easy to identify with what was going on and it felt OK to sit with whatever came up just for that minute: sadness, loneliness, anxiety, or whatever. Somehow, just the intention of pausing and noticing what was going on for me changed things. I started to see if I could pause for another minute . . . and then another, even if I didn't always manage it. Promising myself that I could always go on to eat if it became unbearable. The more I did this, the more often I walked away from food. Just allowing myself to feel for a few minutes meant that I could get on with my life without it. Many times, though, I ended up eating the packet of biscuits knowing that I was using it to soothe myself, but I didn't beat myself up – I knew I would stop eventually. I was doing the best I could and, with time, it kept getting easier to pause and then to stop altogether.

What it boils down to

There are many ways of describing how we use food to cope. Women on our workshops have called it binge eating, overeating, comfort eating, compulsive eating, emotional eating, grazing, bingeing, picking, pigging out, stuffing themselves, treating themselves, overdoing it, indulging, overindulging, constant nibbling, cravings, eating all the time. Call it what you will, it all boils down to the same thing. We call it overeating, because we like the non-judgemental definition. The dictionary definition of overeating is: to eat to excess, especially when habitual. What do you call it? It doesn't matter whether you give it a name or pass it off as an inconsequence, the fact is that so many of us do it and it's not something to be ashamed of. It is simply part of the way we cope.

We all have our different ways of coping with the challenges and emotions of life. For most women it happens to be the same one: food. In fact, we have looked after ourselves the best way we know how; some have chosen more harmful ways of managing and coping: drugs, cigarettes and alcohol, to name but a few.

It's interesting that however differently we describe overeating, we all feel the same way about it: guilty, ashamed, disgusted and out of control. But blaming ourselves for using food in this way is counterproductive. It's easy to tell ourselves that we shouldn't be doing it, that it's unhelpful and destructive. In the long term that may be true, but it is also true that in the short term using food works. It does what we want it to do and our focus is diverted from the feelings or situations we want to avoid whilst experiencing something nice at the same time.

Eating is not an addiction

Using methods that work for other compulsive behaviours such as smoking, drinking, purging (vomiting, laxatives and fasting), drugs, and so on, to stop overeating doesn't work. With all of these we can stop using them forever and avoid tempting situations. We can decide never to light another cigarette, never to have another drink, never to make ourselves sick again. The thing is we can't decide to stop eating forever because we have to eat in order to survive. Nobody can 'give up' food, which is why we need a different approach to deal with using food as a way of managing difficult situations.

One of the most important steps in developing a healthy relationship with food and learning to take care of ourselves without turning to it for comfort and reassurance, is to accept that we do it, first and foremost. Then we need to find out exactly when and how we do it, and then *very slowly*, to allow ourselves to feel whatever it is we would feel, or be however it is we would be, if we were not eating – knowing that emotions don't last forever. Although it can sometimes feel as if we will be overwhelmed by our emotions, the fear of feeling them is often bigger than the actual feeling itself.

Luana R., from London, came on a weekend workshop in London

Before

❝ I would eat to deal with almost any feeling: if I was happy, if I was sad, if I was angry or if I was bored I would eat. When I was happy the food was a celebration, when I was sad it would cheer me up, when I was angry I would use it to stuff the feeling down, and when I was bored it would pass the time. I didn't quite know how I experienced feelings in my body but I knew how to use food to make them go away. Food was my feeling. The feeling I knew very well, though, was the one called guilt, as it seemed to be a constant in my life: guilt for having eaten a "bad" food, guilt for having quit another diet and guilt for having food issues. ❞

Now

❝ After Beyond Chocolate, I became aware of how many feelings I experienced in a day and how many times I used food to help me with those feelings. I began to ask questions: how do I experience feelings? What do they look like? How do they make my body feel? In doing so, I began to understand how they manifested in my body. For example, I learned that anxiety made my stomach churn and my windpipe feel constricted, and I felt fear in my throat with a burning-like sensation. Nowadays I can identify feelings. Instead of eating, I am learning to sit with the feeling and find out what it is like for me. I now ask myself how it feels physically, where I feel it, what thoughts I experienced prior to it, and, slowly, I am using food less to deal with whatever comes up. ❞

Feel it

Putting our feelings and thoughts into words helps us to understand ourselves better. It gives us information and we can then choose when, what and how much we eat. It is difficult to change something that we don't acknowledge. When we tell ourselves it's not OK to feel a certain way we stuff the feelings down with a cup of tea and a packet of biscuits. By allowing ourselves to feel, little by little and with support if we need it, we give ourselves the chance stop eating for comfort or out of habit.

Saying, 'I feel bored, lonely and in need of a treat' gives us more information than saying 'I feel awful' which in turn is more informative than saying I 'I feel urgh!' When we recognise what we are feeling we can allow ourselves to manage without stuffing it all down with food. We can find other ways to manage without always eating to try to make ourselves feel better.

ACTION!

A good place to start:

STOP . . . for 60 seconds.

The next time you get an urge for food, and you know you're not hungry, pause for a minute and tune in before you eat. Make it literally 60 seconds; time it if you want to. You can just sit and think about whatever comes up or you can describe what you are feeling in words. You might not have a clue – it takes practice. Tune in and notice any physical sensations, thoughts and emotions.

1. Close your eyes if you like and then tune into any physical sensations. What do you notice about your body? Do you feel tense, tired, relaxed? Where in your body do you notice these sensations? Is there a tightness in your throat or pressure on your temples? Use as much detail as possible to describe to yourself what you notice about how you feel physically.

2. Next, notice what you are experiencing emotionally. How are you feeling? Sad, happy, angry, fearful? Are you anxious or excited? Bored or lonely?

3. Finally, notice your thoughts. What is going on in your head? What are you thinking about? What are you telling yourself? Are you evaluating, questioning, comparing, criticising, judging, appreciating?

Being specific about your emotions can take practice if you're not used to it. Here is a list of words to use for inspiration. Have a practice now. Tune in and describe what you are feeling as precisely as you can.

Happy

Contented	Satisfied	Excited	Optimistic	Confident
Relaxed	Enthusiastic	Buoyant	Thrilled	Keen
Calm	Grateful	Surprised	Courageous	Light-hearted
Passionate	Loving	Sexy	Interested	Playful

Sad

Ashamed	Discontented	Disappointed	Worried	Weak
Tired	Discouraged	Embarrassed	Lonely	Weary
Gloomy	Vacant	Aching	Pathetic	Bored
Depressed	Tearful	Guilty	Burdened	Melancholy

Angry

Contemptuous	Resentful	Critical	Awkward	Inflamed
Irritated	Enraged	Furious	Annoyed	Irate
Provoked	Offended	Sullen	Indignant	Frustrated
Envious	Cross	Sulky	Bitter	Confused
Grumpy	Boiling	Fuming	Belligerent	Judgemental

Afraid

Powerless	Hesitant	Apprehensive	Nervous	Cowardly
Anxious	Distrustful	Insecure	Suspicious	Cautious
Panicky	Hopeless	Worried	Questioning	Indecisive
Shocked	Tense	Pessimistic	Uncertain	Concerned

What's it like not to eat straight away?

When the minute is up make a choice: you can eat, you can choose not to eat or you can pause for another minute or longer and repeat. Choosing to name our emotions and experience feelings such as boredom, anger, anxiety or sadness instead of distracting ourselves with food can be uncomfortable, but it will pass. In the same way that a packet of crisps or a box of chocolates will eventually finish, no feeling will last forever. You may even discover it was as simple as needing a five-minute break. If the feelings are persistent or particularly strong, find ways of supporting yourself (see Chapter 13). Remember, what you resist, persists.

Notice

Even if you do none of the above, aim to notice as much as you can about when and how you use food. Don't tell yourself to change, just notice. If you normally beat yourself up about it, this time acknowledge that you are using food to help in some way, that you are taking care of yourself the best way you know how to right now, that you are working on making changes – you're just not there yet. Be curious about yourself. Be open to whatever you discover.

Investigate

At the support sessions some participants say they just don't know what they are feeling when they pause and tune in. We turn to food and overeat for many different reasons: this can be anything from a stressful day at the office to a row with a partner or a rainy Sunday morning.

Do you know what triggers you? Investigate and find out;

use a journal if you like writing; the more information you have, the easier it is to make changes.

Pull up a chair

Overeating is often done on the run, standing up in front of the fridge or dipping in and out of packets and pots with repeated trips to the kitchen. Officialising the moment is important: it helps you keep track and focus on what you are feeling and thinking.

We cannot stress this enough: when you put food on a plate and sit down to eat it (this doesn't include in front of the telly) it makes a huge difference. (We will be discussing this important principle in Chapter 6.)

One reason for doing this is to acknowledge that we are eating – not only to ourselves but also to anyone who might see us. When we overeat we often do it in secret. We would be mortified if anyone saw us because we tell ourselves that it's so shameful and disgusting. We all have a right to eat whatever we want, whenever we want it regardless of our shape, size or hunger. We're not suggesting that you shout it out to the world; you don't need an audience, it's just about not hiding.

Other sources of nourishment

Bubble baths, chats with good friends, walks in the park and all those other possibilities are all great things to do that help us feel nourished and good about ourselves. So rather than doing them *instead* of eating, make time for them in your life now, regardless of your eating habits. Allow yourself some undisturbed time in the evening or during your day so that you can nourish yourself in ways that are truly fulfilling and enriching. You don't have to wait until you get the urge to go on a binge to do these things. Make time to do them now.

REALITY CHECK

Creating new habits

By interrupting a repetitive and automatic habit (overeating) and allowing yourself to do things differently, you are giving yourself a chance to create new habits and new ways of responding to recurring problems or emotions. Science has proven that if you exercise your brain beyond your current limits by doing things differently than you are used to, you create new neural pathways.

When you attempt to reach beyond the habitual solutions to a problem (overeating), you are permanently opening new neural pathways in the mind. As you do this regularly, you will create new permanent pathways. Habits of a lifetime take a while to undo, though, so don't get discouraged if this approach doesn't work the first time or even the first ten times. When you learn to tie your shoes, ride a bicycle, drive a car, use a computer keyboard, or learn a musical instrument, your brain gradually develops the neural pathways to make your 'practising' become automatic. The more you practise, and the more quality time you put into your practice, the more your brain pathways change. Fairly soon, tying your shoes or eating when you are hungry becomes automatic and you don't have to think about it any more.

? DID YOU KNOW . . .

Research[1] has shown that snacking when we are not hungry (that is, overeating) does not affect our satiety levels and that people who eat when they are not hungry (whether it's high-carb or high-protein foods) end up eating just as much at the next meal as people who have not snacked.

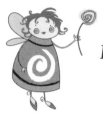

I taste the freedom when . . . I wrap myself in a blanket, not made of chocolate.

Food for thought

- Do you overeat in specific situations?
- Do you overeat at specific times of the day, or month?
- Can you think of any recurrent triggers?

Tune in

Eat when you are hungry

Eat whatever you want

Put it on a plate, sit down and focus

Stop when you are satisfied

Enjoy

Own your body

Move!

Support yourself

Be your own guru

CHAPTER 5

Chocolate sandwiches for breakfast

Consistently depriving ourselves and cutting out certain types of food from our diet ensures we crave them all the more. It is only when we legalise all foods and give ourselves the possibility to eat everything that we can make choices and have a truly healthy approach to weight loss.

Before

I had an obsessive, love–hate relationship with chocolate. I loved it for its sweet, soothing, lusciousness, and hated it for the power it seemed to have over me – the power to make me lose control. It was so hard to eat just one square, and I could easily devour several bars – and often did. I would methodi-cally munch my way through a box of Celebrations in an evening, or stuff them down all in one go on the way home from the supermarket in the car. And then I would feel fat and guilty, and out of control.

Chocolate was one of those foods I considered 'bad' and

thought I shouldn't eat, especially if I was being 'good'. Being good meant being on a diet and eating 'healthy' foods: typically low-calorie, low-fat, low-taste options that would miraculously make me slim. And chocolate wasn't the only culprit. There were many foods that I categorised as bad: cakes, crisps, biscuits, bread, puddings, pastry, cheese, cream, butter and pretty much anything with sugar or fat in it. It never occurred to me that I could eat chocolate or any of those forbidden foods as part of a normal, healthy diet. And although they were officially off-limits, they were the ones I always ended up bingeing on when the going got tough. I never pigged out on salad or carrot sticks. It was the sweet, the stodgy and the creamy I turned to.

The power these foods had over me was so scary that I went to great lengths to avoid them. It was definitely 'all or nothing'. Talk about willpower. I had it by the bucketload. For days, or even weeks, not a morsel of 'bad' food would cross my lips. I would avoid certain aisles at the supermarket, stocking up on vegetables, tofu and low-fat yoghurts. I would manage a few days feeling saintly because I was having a salad at lunch and grilled chicken in the evening. But it was just such hard work. My social life was a maze of potential pitfalls so I avoided meeting up with friends at the pub and refused dinner invitations. I stayed away from restaurants and cafés and generally avoided any situation in which I might be tempted to eat 'bad' food.

Some of the time I felt righteous and very proud of myself, but most of the time I felt miserable and deprived. Eventually I would succumb to the temptation, accept an invitation to dinner, and just one slice of cheesecake was all it took. I had broken the diet, gone off the rails, so I might as well go the whole hog. Then, I would stuff myself with all the delicious sweet and fatty stuff I had missed so much, until tomorrow or maybe Monday, when I would start again, but properly this time.

Now

I eat what I want when I'm hungry. I have no rules about food. I eat an almond croissant and a sweet milky latte for breakfast and cereal for dinner (with a drizzle of cream!). Food has lost its personality; there is no such thing as good food or bad food. Food is just that: food. I am in control; I make the decisions.

I stock a great selection of chocolate in my kitchen cupboards. I have it whenever I fancy it. Most days I have a square or two and I very rarely finish off a bar all in one go (unless it's my dinner!); often, it stays unopened for weeks. If I am hungry for a piece or two, I help myself, sit down and enjoy it and then go back to whatever I was doing. No fuss. And there are days when chocolate is all I fancy and a piece or two is just not satisfying enough. On those days I get a couple of bars out, put some on a plate, enjoy every bite and stop when I've had enough. I know that I can eat it whenever I want to, so there's no temptation to eat it all. If I've had enough after three squares I stop, if it takes the whole bar, or more, no problem.

I have a very balanced diet, without trying hard or making myself eat healthily. I fancy fresh vegetables as often as I fancy chocolate. And on the days when all I fancy is chocolate or crisps or cake, I figure I might be premenstrual or that my blood sugar levels are low or my body needs an energy boost, or simply that I'm in the mood for a particular taste. Whatever the reason: I eat it, I enjoy it and then I move on.

What happened?

I began to realise that the more I resisted these foods and told myself they were bad, the more desperately I wanted them.

Not being allowed to have them was making them all the more attractive. I noticed just how many rules I had about food. How was it that I could hold my ground in a work meeting, fight tooth and nail for a parking spot and generally stick up for myself when I needed to and yet I could be reduced to a quivering wreck in front of a triple-layer chocolate fudge cake?

When I looked closely, I noticed that even when I did eat these forbidden foods, I rarely enjoyed the experience. As I swallowed my first mouthful I was already busy telling myself that I was weak, disgusting and pathetic, and that if I only had a little more moral fibre I wouldn't need to eat them at all. Eating these foods was always accompanied by feelings of guilt, shame and self-disgust.

One day, I took a good look in my kitchen cupboards and saw that there was very little evidence of any of these foods around. I hardly ever bought them as part of the regular shop. Some of the offenders had a place in my home but they were usually there for the children or for my husband. They were 'off-limits' to me and I definitely did not buy them for myself – although that doesn't mean I didn't eat them. They were forbidden after all. I often bought them on the run and ate them hurriedly, in the car or walking home, before they even made it back to my kitchen cupboards. When they did make it that far, I ate them quickly, wolfing them down, and usually standing up in front of the fridge or watching the television.

I realised that because I considered them 'bad', I usually ate them furtively, on my own; the thought of anyone actually seeing me stuffing an entire family-sized packet of chocolate muffins was mortifying. And because I wasn't meant to be eating them, I didn't want any leftovers – they would only remind me of how many calories I had eaten and I just had to get rid of them or I would keep thinking of them until I'd polished them all off. And anyway, I was starting my diet again tomorrow . . .

So I experimented. I let these foods into my life – officially. I decided to make space for the full-fat double cream and the chocolate mousse in my fridge next to the salad and the cottage cheese; to give the peanuts and the crisps their rightful place besides the oatcakes and the Special K in my cupboards. I went out and bought some of my forbidden food, just for myself. I bought *loads*; more than I could possibly eat in one go. I waited until I was hungry and then I gave myself permission to eat. I sat at the table, tasted every mouthful and enjoyed the experience. It was terrifying at first. What if I just couldn't stop and then I ate and ate until I popped?

One of the foods I experimented with was crème caramel. I have always loved it and one helping never seemed quite enough. My favourite is my own home-made version. So instead of making just one family-sized mould, which I know I can wolf down in the blink of an eye, I made three. When I was hungry I took one out, put a good-sized serving on a plate and began to eat slowly. I tasted the silkiness and the richness of the cream. I noticed the burnt sugar in the caramel and the slightly bitter aftertaste. I put my spoon down between each mouthful. When I'd finished the first helping, I paused for a few minutes before deciding if I was still hungry for more. I served another helping and again ate as slowly as I could. It was almost a sensual experience. Two-thirds of the way through the third helping I realised that I had had enough. I paused just long enough (for only about two minutes) to know that I was truly satisfied. And because I knew that I could eat it again whenever I was hungry, it was easy to stop.

For several days I ate nothing but crème caramel and then I went on to chocolate followed by bread and very thickly spread butter. This phase lasted a little while, on and off, and I gradually overcame the fear that I would live off this kind of food for the rest of my life, and that I would never want vegetables again! I learned to trust myself, and to trust that my body would know what was good for me. And as time went by I realised that I was letting go of all those beliefs I had about 'good' and 'bad' foods.

I watched myself make changes – gradually. The more I gave myself permission to eat *anything* when I was hungry, the easier it became to identify what I really wanted. And to my great relief, I found that my body didn't always want chocolate and sweets and cakes and cream as I had feared it would.

What it boils down to

Food is *only* food. It has no personality, and is not intrinsically 'good' or ' bad'. Eating the foods we like when we want them means that we no longer feel the need and desire to have them all the time. If we truly give ourselves permission to eat our forbidden foods whenever we are hungry for them, they lose their power and become ordinary.

In all our workshops most participants react to this idea with horror: 'But that means I'm going to end up eating junk food for months,' they say, or 'That's really unhealthy, what about all the saturated fats and sugars, surely that's bad for me?' We are not suggesting here that it would be fine to have a diet solely made up of KitKats and pizza. Our bodies are so incredibly sophisticated (so much more than any diet doctor) that they naturally ask us for a balanced diet, all food groups included. When given the chance, our bodies crave vegetables and meat as much as chocolate and pizza. The truth is, we eat our forbidden foods anyway, and often we don't realise quite how much of them we eat. So, yes, we might find that for a few months fats and sugars dominate our diet, that all we want are the foods we've told ourselves we shouldn't have, but let's put that in perspective: many of us have spent years and years on failed diets and crazy eating plans, yo-yoing between cabbage soup and Cadbury's – that's hardly healthy. When you listen to your body and respond to its needs you will find that the nutritional quality of your diet will improve. Once you have got it out of your system (and that won't take forever) you will have a lifetime of balanced, healthy eating.

We can only choose *not* to eat when we give ourselves permission *to* eat

We can only tell the difference between foods that we are truly hungry for and foods that we *think* we want, when we give ourselves full permission to eat *all foods*. It is by depriving ourselves of certain foods, by attempting to cut them out of our diets completely, and telling ourselves we shouldn't have them that we step out of balance. How can my body make an informed choice if not *all* the options are available?

Depriving ourselves of these foods or eating them when we think we shouldn't, when we believe that they are bad and fattening, is the surest way to keep craving them and overeating.

One participant came to a workshop thinking that we were going to make her eat so much chocolate that she'd never want to touch it again. Eating whatever we want isn't about having so much of the foods we think are bad or fattening that we will be put off and never want them again. It's about having a balanced diet, not because we are 'trying' to be good but because we really *do* fancy salad and vegetables as much as we fancy chocolate and crisps. We can only do that by knowing that we really can have whatever we want when we want it. When we spend years in that diet mentality, avoiding certain foods and telling ourselves we shouldn't have them, we become like small children. Tell a child that she can't do or have something and she immediately wants it with a vengeance. When we allow ourselves these foods we will find they lose their shine. We may still fancy them but they won't lure us the way they used to. We are as likely to want a hot chocolate and a Danish pastry for breakfast as we are to fancy yoghurt and fruit, and both are equally satisfying. When everything is allowed, we can start to make real choices and have a balanced and healthy diet.

When we give ourselves permission to eat what we want, we can be satisfied and stop when we have had enough. It becomes easier and easier with practice.

When we know that we can eat the foods we love whenever we are hungry for them, we can choose not to eat them when we are hungry for something else: emotional expression, time alone, affection, fun, and so on.

Victoria, from London, came on a weekend workshop in London

Before

❛ Before Beyond Chocolate there were certain foods that I totally banned myself from eating because they would make me fat. Someone had once told me that cheesecake was the most fattening food that you could eat so I hadn't eaten it for ten years. I would crave chocolate everyday mid afternoon. I had a daily battle with myself and I forced myself to eat "healthy" snacks that I didn't enjoy. If I did succumb to my chocolate craving I would feel very guilty and often have a "blow out" that evening. ❜

Now

❝ If I feel like cheesecake, I will go to a fancy deli and buy myself the most delicious slice of cheesecake I can find. I will take it home, put it on a plate and really taste it. Usually, I only want a small amount as I get bored of the taste quite quickly. The power of the cheesecake has gone. I am in control now, cheesecake, schmeezecake! I have a snack drawer at work filled with a wide variety of snacks. If I fancy some chocolate I will eat it. Chocolate bars sit in my drawer for weeks and I forget about them. I can now recognise that sometimes I need a mid-afternoon break rather than sugar. ❞

ACTION!

A good place to start:

Identify your forbidden foods.

List as many as you can think of, being as specific as possible. If your list includes chocolate, for example, is it Cadbury's Dairy Milk or Green & Black's Maya Gold? If it's cheese, can you name a particular type? If it's pasta, is it lasagne? Make your list as long and as detailed as possible, and if you're having trouble figuring out what your forbidden foods are, take a look at the definitions and the list below.

What are forbidden foods?

Forbidden foods are those that you really like but deprive yourself of because you think of them as BAD or FATTENING or UNHEALTHY.

- Forbidden foods are those that you avoid because once you start eating them you can't stop.

- Forbidden foods are those that you treat yourself to or only allow yourself on special occasions.

- Forbidden foods are those that you wouldn't usually eat in front of others.

- Forbidden foods are those that you crave.

- Forbidden foods are those that you eat and then feel guilty about afterwards.

- Forbidden foods are the ones you 'give in' to.

- Forbidden foods are those you buy for other people (your children, your partner, your flatmates) and end up eating anyway.

- Forbidden foods are those that you cannot keep in your cupboards or you won't rest until they're gone.

Examples of forbidden foods

This list is only a very limited assortment; expand and add your own.

Biscuits	Dried fruits and nuts
Bread	Fried foods
Butter	Fruit juice
Cake	Full-fat milk
Cereal	Full-fat yoghurt
Cheese	Hot milky drinks
Chocolate	Mayonnaise
Cream	Pasta
Crisps	Peanuts
Desserts	Pies and pastries

Pizza

Potatoes

Puddings

Salami

Snack bars

Soft drinks

Sweets

Stock up on your forbidden foods

Most diets will tell you not to buy the 'naughty' foods you love. They will advise you to steer clear of those aisles at the supermarket and to say 'no' politely but firmly whenever you are offered a piece of cake or chocolate. Others will tell you that it's OK to have them as a treat, or to save your points for them or to have them in 'moderation' (if only we knew what that meant!). We are about to tell you *exactly the opposite*.

Once you have completed your list, pick *one* of these foods, then go out and by some. Buy lots of it, more than you could possibly eat in one day. We need to be really clear about this. We don't mean three bars of chocolate or six packs of crisps. Loads means at least ten bars of chocolate or 20 packets of crisps (and frankly, if it's within your budget, 20 bars and 30 packs is even better!). The idea is that there is no way you could possibly finish them off before you have a chance to buy some more.

When you are hungry and you fancy that particular food, eat it. Put it on a plate. Make sure there are no distractions when you sit down to eat. Turn off the television or radio and put away books or newspapers. Taste every bite. Enjoy, relish, savour. And when you are satisfied, stop. When you are hungry again, if you want more, have it.

Keep on noticing how you feel about eating this food. Tune in.

◉ Do you enjoy it as much as you thought you would?

◉ Is it delicious?

◉ Is it disappointing?

When you know that *whenever* you want this food, you will have it, it will start to lose its magic power.

Abundance is key

Remember to buy *lots* of this food, if you buy only small quantities you will feel the deprivation before you even start, and it will be tempting to finish it all off, so make sure that abundance rules. You may need to stock up several times in the week to make sure that you always have more than you could eat of whichever food you are buying. Scarcity creates demand. If you think it's running out, you are more likely to finish it all off or feel the need to eat more than you want.

Bianca came to a follow-up session a few weeks ago and told us about the Battenberg cake she had sitting in her kitchen cupboard. 'I can't believe how much is in there. There's tons of it and I don't even want to eat it. I've only had two slices and it's been there since last month. I never imagined that just going out and buying it would make such a difference. I used to polish off a whole cake in one go, I could never get enough of it.'

It's not a treat

You don't have to wait until you have eaten your greens or finished your 'proper meal' before you have your forbidden food, whatever it might be. Have it when you are hungry. It might be hot cross buns or sausage rolls, mashed potatoes or meringues. Whatever it is, allow yourself to have as much as you need to feel satisfied, and *stop* when you have had enough. Remember that you can have this food whenever you want to. The magic of this is that the more you allow yourself to have these foods, the less you will crave them.

Satisfy your cravings

Ignoring your cravings can lead to weight gain. Here's how*: say you fancy a Cadbury's mini roll with your coffee but you tell yourself you shouldn't have it, it's loaded with fat and sugar and you know that each one is a whopping 113 calories. So you decide to be good and you have:

◉ One low-fat digestive biscuit instead (65 calories).

That takes your mind off it for a while. A little later you still fancy that mini roll but you go for something healthy instead:

◉ A handful of nuts and raisins (60 calories).

Throughout the morning you're not really hungry but you still can't stop thinking about food, so you have:

◉ A glass of juice (40 calories),

◉ and some carrot sticks with a low-fat dip (35 calories).

After lunch you're still not satisfied and you just can't resist any longer:

◉ You have a mini roll (113 calories),

* We don't 'do' calories as we know that weight loss and gain is much more complex than a simple calories in/calories out equation. For the sake of illustrating our point in a way that is universally understood, we have made an exception here.

◎ and then another (113 calories),

◎ and then another (113 calories).

Grand total: 539 calories.

And if you think that one mini roll with your coffee wouldn't have satisfied that craving, that's OK . . .
. . . you could have had all three (339 calories). Full stop.

Honest shopping

Get into the habit of honest shopping. Allow these foods into your life officially. They have as much right as the vegetables to be in your trolley with the rest of the shopping. If you buy them in a petrol station with your sunglasses on, you will carry on having 'illicit affairs' with them.

What will people think?

If you're worried about what people will think, remember that a little humour goes a long way. 'I'm feeling a little peckish today' is great way to explain a mountain of Mars Bars to the astonished reaction at the till.

Other people are not half as interested in us as we think they are, the shop assistant is much more likely to be thinking about the next tea break or what's on telly that evening than judging you for buying 30 packs of your favourite crisps. Someone famous once said, 'What other people think of you is none of your business!'

Have them on display

Have an enormous bowl brimming with Smarties on your kitchen table, have a spaghetti jar full of peanuts on your desk, or build a tower of Mars Bars on your coffee table. Replenish often.

Beth, who did a non-residential workshop, used to have a huge bowl of KitKats on her kitchen dresser. She had been known to finish off a family pack in front of the television. To begin with, it needed topping up quite regularly, but over the course of a few weeks she just stopped noticing them, as did the rest of her family. Eventually she put them away because they weren't being touched and she replaced them with another favourite which she had always eaten 'unofficially'.

Mine, mine, mine!

If you live with other people, be they family or flatmates, make sure you have your own shelf for your favourite foods or make it clear that they are yours by labelling them in some way. There's nothing worse than expecting to eat your favourite goodies only to find out that someone else has polished them off.

What are you hungry for?

Tune in and find out. Now that you can eat anything you want, you might find it difficult to identify exactly what it is you are hungry for. When you are hungry and you are not quite sure, close your eyes, tune in and ask yourself if you feel like eating something:

- Hot, cold or at room temperature
- Sweet or savoury
- Crunchy or smooth
- Rich or light
- Spicy or bland

When you have identified something, imagine eating the food that comes to mind, see if you can taste it and notice how it feels once you have eaten it and it is in your stomach.

Will this food satisfy you right now? Remember that in order to identify what you really want, you need to be hungry in the first place, but not too hungry. If you are famished you are much less likely to be able to choose.

It can be fun

Have a forbidden-food night: everyone gets to choose his or her own special favourite. Do it with your children or invite your friends round for dinner with a difference.

REALITY CHECK

In defence of chocolate

Chocolate gets such a bad press; it's accused of all kinds of things, from being addictive and fattening to being downright harmful. This book is not the place for a treatise on chocolate, others have done a wonderful job already, amongst them: Chantal Coady's *Real Chocolate* (Quadrille Publishing, 2004) and Chloé Doutre-Roussel's *The Chocolate Connoisseur* (Piatkus, 2005). What they, along with many others, point out, is that real chocolate is not addictive, fattening or harmful. In fact, according to a study[1] carried out by the Department of Nutrition at the University of California, a bar of real dark chocolate may provide more than just good taste. Substances found in cocoa, called flavinols, may confer benefits such as lowering blood pressure. It is also packed with minerals: 100 grams of dark chocolate contains the following percentages of your daily requirements: 20 per cent iron, 33 per cent magnesium, 27 per cent potassium, 13 per cent calcium. It has to be real chocolate though: made with good quality cocoa beans, a high percentage of cocoa solids and cocoa butter as the only fat. Anything that contains less than 25 per cent of cocoa solids, hydrogenated vegetable fats, lots of refined sugar and a long list of other ingredients and flavourings is *not* chocolate. Most 'commercial' chocolate cannot actually be classified as such according to European directives and yet it is the Mars Bars, the Galaxys, the Celebrations and the After Eights that most women tell us they crave or think they are addicted to. It's not chocolate they crave and overeat. It's a highly palatable concoction of sugar and fat (present in all the above). Women who have been dieting or depriving themselves often do crave fat and sugar, if it's really chocolate you want, then a little goes a long way. Real dark chocolate has such an intense flavour that a few squares does the trick.

Real chocolate isn't hard to come by, you just have to know where to look: Chantal Coady of Rococo, who generously donates lots of chocolate for our workshops, makes some of the best in London. You can visit the King's Road or Marylebone High Street shops or order online. We are working our way through her selection of organic, hand-made bars . . . our current favourite is a 65 per cent dark chocolate with orange and geranium.

If you want to try some fine classics like, Amadei, Bonnat and Domori, log on to www.seventypercent.com and you can even receive a monthly stash. For more places to get real chocolate, see The Chocolate Fairy's favourite resources (p. 219).

? DID YOU KNOW . . .

- We often experience cravings in the evening. This is usually our body's way of demanding a boost. One theory suggests that the amount of carbs we eat impacts on how much serotonin (the feel-good hormone) we produce. If we ignore the craving, our body just shouts louder and louder until it is satisfied. Denying ourselves the food we crave can actually lead to putting on weight.

  Research[2] shows that food cravings are satisfied best by the actual food you are craving – no substitutes will do. As we have said before, the low-fat, low-sugar, low-carb options might fool you for a moment but they cannot fool your body.

- Food cravings can be your body's way of asking for what it needs. This has been scientifically documented. It can happen just before or after your period. A study[3] has shown that in the last week of their menstrual cycle when progesterone levels are high, women experience food cravings because the body needs the extra fuel, and as a result they will eat about 4 per cent more. The fact is that they also burn 4 per cent more calories during the pre-menstrual phase, so it balances out.

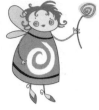

I taste the freedom when . . . half a bar of chocolate stays untouched in the cupboard for days and days and days.

Food for thought

◉ What forbidden food are you going to buy first?

◉ When and where are you going to buy it?

◉ How much are you going to buy?

◉ How do you feel about legalising your forbidden foods?

Tune in

Eat when you are hungry

Eat whatever you want

Put it on a plate, sit down and focus

Stop when you are satisfied

Enjoy

Own your body

Move!

Support yourself

Be your own guru

CHAPTER 6

Eating crisps by candlelight

When we make time to eat with enjoyment and focus, food becomes a delicious, nurturing experience. Why deprive ourselves of this pleasure? Eating with awareness and adopting a few simple, practical strategies is crucial if we want to start when we are hungry, eat the foods we like and know when we've had enough.

Before

I never just ate. I would eat and work, eat and watch television, eat and listen to *The Archers*, eat and tidy the house, eat on the Tube with my nose buried in a book, eat as I walked to the office and eat on the way home. I often ate standing up at the kitchen counter while in a rush to get out of the house, and I regularly gobbled down a sandwich in a cab on my way to a meeting or in front of the computer, because I never seemed to have time for lunch. None of this food ever made it to a plate. Eating a whole pound of cheese in one evening bit by carefully sliced-off bit, with separate trips to the fridge, meant I wasn't really eating a whole pound of cheese. Having a few crackers smeared with butter, meant I was just having a few crackers – even if I eventually finished off the whole packet.

When I did sit down for a meal I could clear the plate in five minutes. I think I learned to eat this fast at boarding school where meals were pretty disgusting and wolfing them down was the only bearable way. I carried on doing this 20 years later, even when the food tasted good. I would get to the last mouthful of bacon and eggs and wonder where it had all gone. I would graze my way through a jumbo packet of tortilla chips in front of the television and be puzzled when my hand rummaged around inside an empty packet. Surely I hadn't eaten all of it already!

When I invited friends over for dinner I would take great care, and get great pleasure from preparing a beautiful meal. I would choose quality ingredients and conjure up some of my favourite dishes. When we sat down to eat I might taste the first bite or two and then I would be worrying about how everyone else was enjoying the food, offering them seconds, bustling in and out of the kitchen. After my guests had left I would pick at the leftovers, sometimes straight from their plates as I was clearing up and feel sorry for myself. Somehow, it felt like I was the only one there who hadn't really enjoyed the food!

Now

Whether it's a four-course meal, a packet of crisps or a few squares of chocolate, I put whatever I am going to eat on a plate, I sit down and taste the food. Whenever I sit at my kitchen table I light a candle before I eat, to remind me to eat slowly and mindfully. I put my knife and fork down between mouthfuls, and I am so practised now that when I have friends round to dinner I can have a laugh and still enjoy the food.

I make time to eat even when I'm rushed off my feet. I stop whatever I am doing and put everything on hold, even if it's only for ten minutes. By eating slowly I give my body the time it needs to send satisfaction signals to my brain and register that I've had enough. It also means that, often, one chocolate or a small portion is enough to satisfy me and my taste buds.

What happened?

I stopped eating in front of the television, I switched off the radio and put away the newspaper and just sat there: me and my food. It felt very strange and quite a challenge to start with. I had been so used to distracting myself that focusing solely on the food was uncomfortable and unfamiliar. I was so good at taking myself away from the experience of eating that if at first there were no distractions, I'd just daydream.

Very gradually, though, I was able to focus for a little longer each time. I made a point of always sitting down to eat; I would put the food on a plate and eat as slowly as I could. Really tasting the food was a revelation. I discovered that there were some foods I had been eating for years that I found really rather unpalatable and others that I had eaten without enthusiasm that tasted quite delicious when I paid attention. As I slowed my pace, the food became more satisfying and enjoyable. I stopped eating on the go and made time for meals and snacks.

The more I focused on the food the more dissatisfying it became to eat when I wasn't hungry. Sitting down to eat and focusing my attention on the food felt like an important way of telling myself that it was OK to give myself a break, to satisfy my needs and desires and to enjoy the pleasures of eating what I want.

What it boils down to

By putting the food on a plate, sitting down and eating without all the usual distractions we are giving ourselves a chance to really slow down. This makes it so much easier to eat when we are hungry, to know when we are satisfied and to decide what we want to eat. It also makes it easier to stop overeating. By officialising the moment, we can avoid the mindless grazing or intermittent picking that we do when we're not really hungry.

In the end it's all about giving ourselves time to celebrate something that we have to do every single day of our lives.

Pam Curtis, from Dorset, did the multimedia course

Before

⁶ When I came home after picking my children up from school, the first thing I did was go to the snack cupboard. It was a habit really, I wasn't hungry. I could quite easily eat three, four or even five packets of crisps without noticing. I hid the packets from my children, eating in secret, hoping nobody would notice how many snacks I had taken. I would eat them so quickly that by the time I had eaten the last packet, I couldn't remember tasting *any* of the crisps. When I was finished eating, I usually felt unsatisfied and guilty. This habit was repeated regularly. ⁹

Now

❝ I buy nice, speciality crisps in big bags. When I am hungry and feel like some, I take a bowl from the cupboard and put a handful in. I sit at the table and enjoy every single crisp. I eat them slowly, and I can definitely taste the amazing flavours. For me, this is a very satisfying way to eat crisps and I am happy to eat fewer. I don't need to raid the cupboard as soon as I walk in, I know they are there for when I am ready to enjoy them. The guilt has been replaced with pleasure and satisfaction. ❞

ACTION!

A good place to start:

Put it on a plate.
Putting food on a plate interrupts the hand-to-mouth action of dipping in and out of packets that many of us don't even notice until it's too late. By using a plate, you officialise the fact that you are eating. You can't pretend that you are not. You give yourself the chance to decide how much food to take; you don't have to finish the bag or the packet. Whatever you eat, put the food on a plate first, even if it's a sandwich, a bar of chocolate or a packet of crisps. By putting it on a plate you bring your attention to the food. This is always possible – keep some paper plates in your office drawer.

Sit down

It can seem such a waste of time to do nothing but eat, and yet, by setting aside a moment to sit down and eat without distractions, it's amazing what a different experience eating can be. Sitting down makes it easier to focus. When you can, lay the table. It doesn't have to be a dining table, you could sit on a stool at the kitchen counter or eat off a tray or at your coffee table in the sitting room. The title of one of our favourite books by Geneen Roth says it perfectly: *When You Eat at the Refrigerator, Pull Up a Chair.*

One-minute transition

Often, when we sit down to a meal we start eating immediately without taking the time to acknowledge that we have stopped whatever we are doing and are starting a new activity: eating. Before you start, take just one minute to leave behind whatever it is you were doing and bring yourself to the meal or snack you are about to have. Take a few deep breaths and tune in, become aware of any physical sensations, thoughts or feelings. How hungry are you? Is the food on your plate what you really want? Lighting a candle before you sit down to eat, or finding another way of marking the transition, is a helpful way to remind you to do this.

Slow food

Bernadette came to a support session one evening and told us how she had been having microwaved WeightWatchers' lasagne for months, sitting in front of the television, eating it straight from the plastic container it came in. When she put it on a plate, sat down at the table and focused, she realised that it tasted horrible; she found it really rather revolting. She had been eating it once a week and hadn't even noticed. She never had one again.

Put your knife and fork down between mouthfuls rather than preparing the next one whilst you're still chewing. If you are eating a sandwich, put it down between bites. Eat one crisp at a time, slowly. Experiment. See just how slowly you can eat and then find a pace that works for you; one that allows you to taste the food properly without it feeling like a chore at every meal. Eat a Western meal with chopsticks to slow yourself down and focus (not recommended with peas). We are not suggesting you eat every meal at a snail's pace, rather that you adopt 'slow food' as a general attitude.

Focus

Our attention needs to be on the food, to notice the way it looks, the way it smells and the way it tastes. When we wolf it down in a few mouthfuls, distracted by the television or rushing and grabbing something on the go, we are more likely to overeat because we miss out on the experience altogether. Eating is a life-sustaining activity that deserves your time and attention.

When you eat . . . just eat!

Do away with distractions. Switch off the television or the radio, put down what you are reading and put the heated, distracting conversations on hold until you have finished.

Enjoy

Food can be a delicious, nurturing, sensual experience. Why deprive ourselves of this pleasure? Make each meal a feast.

Invite yourself to dinner

Choose a pretty tablecloth or placemat. If you have any fancy china or crystal glasses, now is the time to use them. Make your mealtime special, lay the table, light a candle, cut a few flowers from your garden and put them in a little vase. Bon appétit!

Yes, but . . . no, but . . . I can't do all that!

If you're thinking that you can't possibly do all of these things every time you eat, then don't! Take one that you think you can manage and decide that you will set aside one mealtime to do it. See what works for you. Do one thing at a time.

REALITY CHECK

Beyond Chocolate goes Zen!

Although we recommend a one-minute transition – taking a few breaths and tuning in before you eat – it would never cross our minds to suggest meditating before a meal, that's not really up our street. Imagine our surprise when we discovered a scientific study on Eating-Specific Mindfulness Meditation[1]. The study shows that meditation leads to less bingeing and overeating, feeling less depressed and anxious around food, as well as feeling more in control of eating and awareness of hunger and satiety cues. And guess how they did it? Participants were instructed to, and we quote, 'take a few moments to stop and become aware of thoughts and feelings, at times such as prior to meals . . . take note of whatever thoughts, emotions, or bodily sensations arise, returning attention to the breath when it engages with another focus'[2]. Maybe meditation is our thing after all. We call it tuning in and it only takes one minute . . . and we always thought you had to meditate with your legs crossed, sitting on the floor doing your best not to think about anything at all!

? DID YOU KNOW . . .

The story about the monk who came across one of his students eating his meal while reading a book? The master took the book away and snapped it shut saying, 'When you eat, eat and when you read, read.' The very next day the student saw the monk eating his meal under a tree with his nose in a book. 'Master!' he exclaimed, 'only yesterday you said when you eat, eat and when you read, read. I don't understand . . .'

'Yes,' replied the monk, 'and when you eat and read, eat and read.'

If you enjoy eating without distractions and know that you will do it, all well and good. If you find it a challenge, then experiment with keeping your focus on the food even if you are doing something else. Put it on a plate, sit down and focus as much as you can. Notice how doing something changes the way you taste or enjoy the food, and if it means you eat more, less or the same.

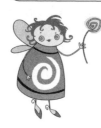

I taste the freedom when . . .
every grape is a feast.

Food for thought

- How do you distract yourself when you eat?

- How often do you notice the subtle differences in the texture and taste of food?

- How can you remind yourself to focus?

Tune in

Eat when you are hungry

Eat whatever you want

Put it on a plate, sit down and focus

Stop when you are satisfied

Enjoy

Own your body

Move!

Support yourself

Be your own guru

CHAPTER 7

Just how much is enough?

Knowing when to stop and being happy to do so is vital to weight loss. Overeating is overeating, even if it's carrots! If you are hungry to start with and you listen carefully, your body will let you know when to stop. But just how much is enough? Enough is about eating until you are satisfied, and feeling satisfied is not necessarily the same as feeling full.

Before

When I sat down to my bowl of pasta for dinner, I thought that the right time to stop was when it had all gone or, if I had cooked enough for a family of four, 'enough' meant when I was stuffed to bursting. I would really enjoy the first couple of mouthfuls and then I would look down and the bowl would be empty and I couldn't remember eating any of it so I had to go back for seconds and start all over again. When I was on the latest diet or following some self-imposed plan, it wasn't up to me anyway, but invariably those meagre portions were never enough.

When I was off the diet I was eating for Britain and the rest of Europe. Sometimes I grazed all day: biscuits with my tea in the morning, and again in the afternoon, a packet of crisps at my desk at mid morning, a bar of chocolate on the Tube, and on and on, peanuts while I cooked dinner and repeated visits to the kitchen cupboard for chocolate wafers and wine gums while I watched television. On and on ... until by late evening I was totally stuffed. I felt full, but not satisfied. I would force myself to eat the steamed carrots and grilled fish I thought I should have for dinner but it was never enough. It wasn't that I was hungry – I just felt a compelling need to eat. So, after my healthy meal, I would end up munching on those chocolate wafers and sucking on the wine gums until bedtime. I didn't even taste the food. As I ate it quickly without thinking, usually furtively so that I wasn't giving myself a chance to appreciate it, there was no way I could feel satisfied. I remember one night staying at my parents'. As I prowled around the house looking for something sweet I stumbled on a box of After Eights my mum had bought to pass round after her dinner party the next evening and I thought I would have one or two – there would still be more than enough left for the next day. The problem is I told myself that quite a few times, every time I went back for a couple more. I wanted to keep the box looking intact, so I left the little wrappers inside and slipped the chocolates out. At one point, rummaging through the wrappers to find another one, I realised there was not a single chocolate left. I was horrified! I had eaten my way through an entire box of After Eights and I *still* wanted more!

Now

I eat as much as it takes to satisfy me. Satisfaction comes in different forms: it might mean a five-course meal in a fabulous restaurant that leaves me groaning; savouring one particular dish; or having just a little of something. One or two squares of chocolate can do the trick, I don't need the whole bar. I eat only the foods that I really want, and if this means having risotto for breakfast, so be it. I do not control my portion sizes and if this means needing two avocados at lunch, then that's OK, too. Knowing that I can always eat again as soon as I am hungry means that I am quite happy to leave food on the plate or in the packet. In fact, stopping when I'm satisfied rather than full up usually means that I will be hungry again sooner . . . and I get to eat again!

I have no rules and no routine. Every day is different. I listen to what my body tells me and stop eating when I am truly satisfied, not when I think I ought to or should. Last but not least, I have never put the weight I lost back on, despite the creamy risottos and bars of chocolate for breakfast.

What happened?

I started tuning in to physical sensations when I ate and learned to recognise the signals. I found it hard, really hard. I had spent so many years dieting that I didn't know how much was enough because I was either being 'good' and having to go hungry or being 'bad' and stuffed to the brim. So I experimented with stopping when I felt that I had had enough of whatever I was eating. This was really tricky at first.

Somehow I went from still feeling hungry and wanting more to being full up and bursting without noticing. It was hard to leave food on my plate; it was even harder not to order dessert at the restaurant, even if I was quite full. Over the months, however, I learned to recognise the different levels that lead from hungry to satisfied. Suddenly instead of only 'stuffed' or 'starving' I had four levels in between. I had never thought about the difference between full and satisfied, and it certainly never occurred to me that I could be satisfied and stop eating without feeling full.

I realised that until I understood what truly satisfied me, rather than what merely filled me up I would never break away from the diet mentality that kept me controlling portion sizes and still checking on *how much* I was eating. I could see that being willing to stop, depended on a lot more than feeling full. When I started eating because I was hungry and I ate what I really fancied, slowly, enjoying it and tasting every mouthful, it was so much easier to know just how much was enough.

What it boils down to

We are born knowing exactly how much nourishment we need and when we need it. The truth is our body knows; it has been designed to give us clear signals so that we can tell when we are hungry and when we have had enough to eat. There's a very good reason for this. By eating just how much we are hungry for, we make sure that our body is receiving the amount of energy it needs – no more, no less. Not only is this more satisfying it is also healthier for our bodies and is essential for long-term weight loss.

There's no set point at which to stop eating. It changes from day to day and depends on many different factors: from how you are feeling, to what you are eating to what your plans are for the day. And portion sizes aren't a measure either. A portion size is totally arbitrary – it is decided by product managers and marketing teams, doctors and experts who have no idea how much we're going to be hungry for at any given time. Being able to stop when you've had enough depends on both physical and emotional satisfaction. Over the years of being told how much to eat by others, we forget how to tune in and listen to the messages our body gives out and we lose awareness. We also start believing that we are bottomless pits, that there will never be enough and that we will never be satisfied.

Focus on satisfaction

A little while after attending a weekend workshop, Bella sent us an email saying, 'So far I have become good at tasting every morsel that goes into my mouth. I am finding that the longer I take and the more I savour, the less I need to eat. So far so good.' Being satisfied and knowing that we have had enough isn't the same as being full. To be truly satisfied so that we can stop eating and leave food we don't want, we have to be willing to trust ourselves, to trust that we will look after ourselves by eating when we are hungry and eating the foods we like, and trusting that we will know when we have had enough and are truly satisfied.

Caroline Johnson-Marshall, from London, came on a weekend workshop in London

Before

❝ I was so focused on food I ate without being hungry all the time, as if the food would not be available if I didn't eat it straight away. So I'd down it without thinking. It was as if I was afraid of waiting to be hungry; the anxiety would be too much. The anxiety would "eat me up"! I ate to make sure I wouldn't get hungry. ❞

Now

❛ I feel like I'm really imbibing the principles of Beyond Chocolate at a deep level so my behaviour is changing. I have noticed myself recently saying "NO, wait until you're hungry." And then I think of all the wonderful foods that I will really taste and enjoy (it's a lot to do with love and self-esteem). I make sure that I have a nice selection of my favourite goodies to choose from. Having the wonderful "secrets" of eating consciously and stopping at enough, eating whatever I want, anything at all, means that I don't need to be jealous of people who eat what they want and don't get fat, because I can do that too if I focus on my delicious self! Beyond Chocolate has been life-changing and such a precious gift. ❜

ACTION!

A good place to start:

What are your different levels of satisfaction?

In the same way that you assess how hungry you are before you eat, it can be very useful to tune in and get a sense of how satisfied you feel when you stop. This will then enable you to make decisions about when and how much food you want to eat. Use the 0 to 5 scale on page 42 to build up a picture.

Describe the physical sensations, thoughts and emotions connected to each level of satisfaction.

Full or satisfied?

Pick a meal to experiment with – sitting at the table, in a comfortable and relatively calm environment. Aim to notice if there is a difference between feeling full and being satisfied. Every so often put your knife and fork down and tune in. Notice all the sensations, feelings and thoughts connected to fullness. Notice the subtle changes as you begin to feel fuller.

◉ How much food does it take for you to feel full?

◉ Decide when you want to stop.

◉ Are you satisfied?

Do it again at another meal but this time, focus on how satisfied you feel.

◉ How much food does it take for you to feel satisfied?

◉ Decide when you want to stop.

◉ Are you full?

Just like your hunger, you can begin to build up a picture of your different levels of satisfaction. There is no right place to stop. You decide.

Be hungry when you start eating

If you are not hungry in the first place you are unlikely to be able to recognise the signals that help you decide when to stop. When you are eating to satisfy an emotional hunger, there can never be enough food – to feel satisfied you will need to give yourself whatever you are truly hungry for.

Know that you can eat again whenever you are hungry

If you think that this is your last chance to eat any particular food or your last chance to eat whatever you like before you start that diet on Monday or next week, or the month before your holiday, you will eat to defend against the deprivation to follow.

Create your own portions

When it comes in a bag or a pack, it's so easy to cram a few more in to finish it off or simply to eat a whole portion, because it's a portion. So, instead of opening one packet of biscuits at a time, open three or four and empty them into a tin. Then you can decide exactly how many you want to eat. This is especially useful for things that come in 'handy portion sizes', such as crackers, sweets in boxes, crisps, nuts, biscuits and loads more. It is much easier if *you* are in control of how much food you put on your plate. Only you know the size of the portion that you need, so make it easier for yourself to decide by storing food in larger quantities than you could eat in one go and investing in a good set of plastic boxes with lids, jars and tins. That way you decide when to stop rather than waiting until there's none left.

Whenever possible ask to help yourself to food. Other people don't know how hungry you are and how much you will need to feel satisfied.

Eat what you want

If you are eating certain foods because you think they are good for you or will help you lose weight because they are low in calories, or fat, or carbs, you may feel physically full but you will not be satisfied. You will be left wanting more and eating more. And when we tell ourselves that the low-fat, low-sugar, low-carb, low-*taste* options are better because we can eat more of the foods we like, we may fool ourselves for a moment, but we don't fool our bodies. If your body is expecting sugar, it won't be satisfied by an aspartame substitute.

Put it on a plate

If you eat out of a packet you won't be giving yourself the chance to gauge how much you need and it will be that much more difficult to notice when you reach satisfaction.

Eat slowly

It can take up to 15 minutes or even longer for your stomach to communicate to your brain that you have had enough food, so if you eat too quickly you will miss the signals altogether.

Focus

To be able to stop, you have to be eating consciously. When you are eating without distractions (without the television, radio, books, and so on) it's so much easier to be aware of your body's signals and to make a choice to stop when you have had enough.

Half-time

Eat half the food on your plate and tune in to see what level of satisfaction you have reached. You might start out with the best of intentions and then find yourself forgetting to tune in after a few minutes. Finding ways to remind yourself can help you to stay focused.

Be willing to waste food

Stopping when you are satisfied means not feeling compelled to finish every scrap on your plate. It means being willing to put food away, throw it away or give it away. If you're a member of the clean-plate club, experiment with different portion sizes: start small, you can always go back for more.

REALITY CHECK

What is a portion anyway?

When you go to a restaurant, do you usually polish off every morsel of food that is on your plate? Have you ever stopped to think about how much food will satisfy you? We asked ourselves if restaurants follow some kind of universal rule regarding portion sizes and came across a fascinating study that looked at the changes in portion sizes in the US between 1977 and 1998[1].

Not surprisingly, the study showed that portion sizes had increased noticeably. The problem is that when we are presented with more food on a plate than we need to satisfy our hunger, most of us will eat more without even thinking about it. After all, most people eat what they are given, especially when the food is good, which it should be in a restaurant.

The good news is that we found another study[2] showing that although we eat more when given larger portions, we still feel satisfied when given less. This is proof that quantity is not necessary for satisfaction. We can be satisfied with less food.

In this study, customers at a restaurant were given different serving sizes of the same pasta dish. The portion served varied between a standard serving and a serving 50 per cent larger. Customers who ordered the meal were asked to rate their satisfaction and the appropriateness of the portion size.

The results showed that customers who were served the larger portion ate nearly all of it but that *all* the customers rated the size of their portions as appropriate for meeting their needs.

So the next time you go out for a meal, stop and think: how much of the food on your plate do you need to satisfy your hunger?

? DID YOU KNOW . . .

When we eat food that contains fat, the intestine releases a hormone called cholecystokinin. This hormone is the chemical messenger that responds to fat and it is responsible for communicating to the brain that we are getting near satisfaction. Researchers[3] found that the women whose meals were higher in fat experienced greater feelings of satiety and had significantly higher cholecystokinin responses than the women who were given low-fat, low-fibre meals. In layman's terms this means that if we avoid fat or favour low-fat options we are less likely to be satisfied and therefore to know when to stop.

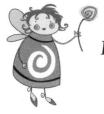

I taste the freedom when . . . I start with the pudding and have a main course if I'm not satisfied.

Food for thought

◉ How do you know when you are satisfied?

◉ How do you decide when you have had enough?

◉ When do you stop?

◉ Is it easy to leave food?

◉ How much is a portion?

CHAPTER 8

You are not a dustbin

Stopping when you are satisfied and eating whatever you want may mean leaving food uneaten on your plate or in the fridge. There are many ways to avoid wasting food that don't involve eating it.

Before

I've never had much of an issue with throwing food away, probably because of the attitudes I was brought up with. My father couldn't bear to eat leftovers and my mother threw anything that hadn't been eaten after a meal straight into the bin. The starving children in Africa were never mentioned. While I sometimes felt uncomfortable with the idea of so much good food going to waste, I didn't actually feel compelled to eat it. Having said that, I wasn't beyond finishing off a tasty cake because it would be a shame to see it go to waste, and I usually cleaned my plate in restaurants – I didn't know when I would have the chance to eat that food again and I had paid an arm and a leg for it. I wasn't about to waste even one a precious morsel. I could never bring myself to leave half an uneaten prawn and avocado sandwich – they were just too good.

I used to cook enough pasta to feed my family and the family next door. I was afraid that if I didn't make loads there wouldn't be enough for *me*. There was something comforting about having masses of food available. My husband would eat more than he really wanted to avoid the waste and I'd scrape the rest it into the bin systematically, feeling a bit guilty and ashamed. Every week I bought lots of gorgeous organic fresh vegetables, fruit and salads at the supermarket and so much of it would rot away at the bottom of the fridge while I delved repeatedly into the biscuit tin. The result was that I spent lots of money on food but much of it ended up in the bin.

Now

Since I've started running workshops and meeting women for whom it is a significant issue, I see waste in a different light. I have come up with lots of creative and acceptable ways to make sure that I waste as little food as possible. Eating it is not an option. I've become really good at gauging how much food I need to shop for (learned through trial and error) and now I cook in relation to everyone's appetites. I know there will be enough for me and if there isn't I'll know for next time and I can always make a bit more or have something else. If I've misjudged it and there's food left over, I find someone who will appreciate it: a friend or neighbour or a colleague – or the guy sitting on the floor at the Tube station (he was very pleased with my spare slice of chocolate cheesecake a few weeks ago). And I'm tickled pink by the new Slim Pret – a half sandwich from Pret a Manger – because it means I can have my favourite sandwich and I am still hungry for the slice of carrot cake.

What happened?

When I started running Beyond Chocolate workshops I realised that what for me had not been a problem, was a major issue for most women. The issue of waste seemed to come up over and over again. Women couldn't stop eating when they were satisfied because they didn't know what to do with the leftovers. Their beliefs about wasting food took many different forms and all had the same outcome: they ate food that they didn't necessarily want or need because they couldn't bring themselves to waste it. If they threw it away they would be disregarding all those starving children in Africa, disrespecting their parents' experiences of rationing during the war, throwing money down the drain, and so on. By not eating something because they didn't want it they felt that they were being too frivolous, selfish, thoughtless or pandering to a whim.

I began to see that to nourish ourselves would mean finding creative and acceptable ways of dealing with the waste as well as challenging some of our outdated beliefs. On one of our very first workshops, as we were discussing whether it was better to throw food away or eat it, Babette, an incisive and witty participant, piped up 'I'm not a dustbin!'. That's when it all fell into place – with that one comment. It clicked, whether I throw it in the bin or into my body, if it's not wanted or needed, it's wasted anyway.

What it boils down to

Excess food will turn to waste either inside our body or outside it. If we eat to avoid wasting it, then we are treating ourselves like a dustbin.

When we are willing to stop when we are satisfied and find ways of dealing with leftovers we treat our body with the respect and kindness it deserves and are taking another step towards permanent weight loss.

When we tell ourselves that the right thing to do is to finish what's on our plate, to polish off what's left of the tiramisu in the fridge or to force down a slice of congealed pizza, what we are actually saying is that it's OK for us to be the dustbin. Throwing it in the bin is just wrong, but throwing it into our body is fine.

Now it's time to update our beliefs about waste. It's certainly not by eating that we are going to help the starving children in Africa. Nowadays, far from being rationed and scarce, there is a nauseating overabundance of food in the Western world; *we* will not go hungry. Messages about how wrong it is to waste food and others like them have been passed down to us for generations. By revising our attitudes to waste and food in general we can ensure that future generations don't inherit these unhelpful beliefs.

We can find ways to avoid creating waste in the first place, and when there is food left over there are plenty of ways to deal with it, apart from throwing it in the bin.

Louise, from London, came on a retreat in Puglia, Italy

Before

❝ No matter how full I felt, I always finished my plate, or even ate the leftovers from the saucepan rather than throw food away. I would do this hurriedly, even if no one was in the house, almost like throwing food into a bin. ❞

After

❝ I no longer feel guilty about throwing food into the bin, or leaving food on the plate either when eating at home or in a restaurant. Although "your body is not a waste bin" is a simple statement, as a concept it was a revelation. ❞

ACTION!

A good place to start:

Update your beliefs about waste and redefine the ways in which you approach it.

Take a piece of a paper and make a list of beliefs you have or messages that you grew up with about waste.

Example:
I must finish all the food on my plate because there are children starving in Africa.

When you have come up with as many as you can think of, look back over what you have written. Ask yourself the following questions about each one:

1. Is it helpful?

2. Is it out of date?

3. How does it limit me?

4. Do I really believe it?

5. Would eating the food really make a difference?

6. Is this my belief or does it belong to someone else?

7. Do I want to keep it or let it go?

Tear or cut the paper into strips so that you have one belief on each piece.

Make a pile of all the beliefs and attitudes you would like to let go of. Tear them up into little pieces and throw them in the bin.

continued

If you find it hard to let go of your beliefs about waste and you're still eating, don't beat yourself up – you're not a punchbag either. It can take time to change old habits, so be kind to yourself.

Intelligent shopping 1: more is less

Go shopping several times a week rather than doing one large weekly shop. You're more likely to buy the food you really fancy and reduce the likelihood of food going off in the fridge untouched. When you are buying a small amount of food and you know what you want, it is usually a much quicker and less thankless task.

Intelligent shopping 2: two in one

If you are too busy to go to the supermarket more often, do your shopping at lunchtime and kill two birds with one stone: a walk as well as providing for your evening meal all in one go.

Intelligent shopping 3: embrace new technology

Internet shopping can be a godsend if you are busy or have small children. It also means that you will really think about what you want rather than making impulse buys.

Honest shopping

Another benefit of buying the foods you like and are actually going to eat is that you will have less waste. No more mouldy salads at the bottom of the fridge or uneaten rice cakes going stale in the cupboard.

Little by little

When you help yourself to food, take a smaller amount to begin with and help yourself to more if you are still hungry. Not because you should be eating less but because it's easier to decide when to stop without leaving food on the plate. If you have a family or live with someone else, put food in serving dishes and let everyone help themselves rather than serving all the food up on to everyone's plate straight from the pan. If you have children, you'll be teaching them a valuable skill, learning to recognise how much food they are hungry for.

Be creative

If you do have food left over that you don't want, find a way of using it that feels appropriate to you: give it to someone who would like it (a homeless person, a neighbour, colleague, the dog, the compost heap).

Freeze some for another day when you will feel like eating it again, store it in the fridge if it will keep for a day or two, and if you still haven't eaten it by then, throw it away. Find ways that work for you.

REALITY CHECK

How waste turns to fat

Do you know what happens to that slice of congealed pizza if you eat it instead of putting it in the bin?

1. You chew the food and your saliva starts to break down the starch into sugar.

2. You swallow it down, and the sugar, fat and water are churned up in your stomach where it is broken down even more and turned into a substance called chyme.

3. It enters your duodenum (the first part of your small intestine that connects to the stomach), where your gall bladder secretes the digestive juice bile.

4. The bile dissolves the fat, making it easier to absorb.

5. Meanwhile, your pancreas (the gland behind your stomach) is busy secreting enzymes into your duodenum to break down the sugar, fat and protein even further.

6. Now your pizza is a nice thin liquid, and it's ready to be absorbed through the lining of the small bowel. Fat, sugar and protein wave goodbye to each other and go their separate ways.

7. The sugar goes straight into your bloodstream, supplying various organs on the way. Whatever is left over is converted to fat and stored in fat cells.

8. The fat also goes straight into your bloodstream. Your liver works its magic, burning some of it and converting the rest into various substances such as cholesterol. What's left over is reunited with the sugar in your fat cells where they both settle down comfortably until they're needed.

9. The protein needs a little more work before it can enter the bloodstream: it is broken down into peptides, and then into amino acids.

10. The amino acids enter your bloodstream through the lining of your small intestine.

11. Some of the amino acids feed your muscles; what's left over converts to fats and sugars, and joins the club in your fat cells.

No matter what you eat, your body sends whatever it can't use to your fat cells. So chuck the leftover slice of pizza into the bin, not into your fat cells.

 DID YOU KNOW . . .

The Collins Dictionary definition of waste: to use, expend or consume thoughtlessly, carelessly or to no avail. Sounds like eating food you are not hungry for to us.

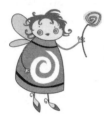 *I taste the freedom when . . . I resign my membership of the clean-plate club.*

Food for thought

- When was the last time you ate something rather than throwing it away?
- How was waste dealt with when you were growing up?

Tune in

Eat when you are hungry

Eat whatever you want

Put it on a plate, sit down and focus

Stop when you are satisfied

Enjoy

Own your body

Move!

Support yourself

Be your own guru

CHAPTER 9

Eating chocolate, without the guilty aftertaste

We spend so much time worrying guiltily about food and what we have or haven't eaten that we often forget how enjoyable it can be. Bringing back enjoyment, pleasure, fun and lightness to our relationship with food . . . *and* our bodies, is one of the best parts of life Beyond Chocolate.

Before

It's surprising how little I enjoyed food, considering how much and how often I thought about it. Food and eating brought up lots of feelings, and joy was rarely one of them! I felt guilty when I ate 'bad' foods that were supposed to be off-limits, or depressed and frustrated when I had to say no and settle for 'being good'. Sometimes I would enjoy the first mouthful of a chocolate bar, but that was soon clouded by the guilt of having eaten something fattening. I often felt panicky and confused: how many calories were in that muffin? What was the fat content in that brunch? Did that low-fat yoghurt count as one or two portions? Was it OK to have the jacket potato with tuna or was that mixing carbs and protein?

Sometimes I even felt disgusted: with myself as I carried on eating way past the 'bursting, need to lie down' phase or when trying to convince myself that the nauseating, chalky liquid I was about to have for lunch *did* taste of strawberry. I might enjoy a great meal out or special dinner my mum had cooked for me, but it was always tinged with guilt and the knowledge that I'd eaten too much.

I certainly didn't enjoy anything much about my body. I didn't enjoy flailing my arms about in step classes and I didn't enjoy trying to squeeze myself into a pair of jeans that were a size too small. I felt guilty and depressed getting dressed in the morning, as I rummaged through clothes that didn't fit. There was nothing enjoyable about looking in the mirror and it certainly wasn't fun comparing myself to the models in the magazines.

Now

Each meal is a feast. Whether I'm eating a square of chocolate, a packet of Walker's cheese and onion crisps, scrambled eggs on toast or a Sunday roast with all the trimmings, I thoroughly enjoy the experience. I go out of my way to track down my favourite foods: a particular type of bread (sourdough raisin and hazelnut) or the white chocolate saffron and cardamom truffles from Rococo. When I go out and discover a dish I love, I have fun experimenting with dozens of different recipes until I manage to make it for myself, just so. Food has become an enjoyable part of my life, and eating produces sighs of pleasure rather than guilty groans. When I move my body I do it for pleasure as well as for my health. I know jogging, dancing, walking, yoga and swimming are good for me but, just as importantly, that's how I enjoy moving. I plan my shopping trips so that they will be fun and satisfying, rather than exhausting and depressing.

What happened?

As I started to make changes to my relationship with food and my body, I started to enjoy things a lot more. Eating when I was hungry was so much more enjoyable than eating when I wasn't. By tuning in I gradually found it easier and easier to decide exactly what and how much would satisfy my taste buds, which meant eating became a pleasure rather than aimlessly picking or forcing unappetising low-taste options on myself. I also noticed how often feelings of guilt stopped me from enjoying food. It was always when I thought I shouldn't be eating something, when I was eating to please others or when I thought I definitely should be eating something else, something healthier or less fattening, that I felt guilty. So every time I caught myself thinking this way, I reminded myself that by eating whatever I wanted, I would feel less compelled to eat just because it was there or because I felt deprived.

I allowed myself to eat all my forbidden foods and taste them properly for the first time. That's when I discovered I didn't even like most of the chocolate I had been eating! It was too sweet and too cloying. I started to look for alternatives and discovered *real* chocolate; suddenly my Achilles heel became the most pleasurable of hobbies. The more I ate out of physical hunger and stopped when I was satisfied, the less guilty I felt – even when I was eating bread and thickly spread butter! Every time I fancied a packet of fizzy cola bottles, I reminded myself to eat them slowly, one at a time, and, rather than scoffing a pack down guiltily in a few frenzied minutes, I found that a few eaten slowly were quite enough. No guilt trip needed.

I realised that in fact I felt guilty about pretty much anything to do with my body: from my weight (I was too heavy) to exercising (I wasn't doing enough) and all those chocolate bars in between. I stopped doing things that I knew induced guilt, such as counting calories, reading the diet pages in the magazines (actually I stopped reading the glossies altogether!) and weighing myself every morning on the bathroom scales. I started doing things that were fun instead. I had a party with a massive tower of home-made profiteroles drowned in hot chocolate sauce, which sent the guests into frenzied delight. I started jumping around my living room to my favourite music, working up a sweat worthy of the most gruelling step class. I treated myself to some really gorgeous underwear that fitted properly. Gradually, by integrating all the Beyond Chocolate principles into my life, I began to enjoy life more and more.

What it boils down to

When we eat with enjoyment and pleasure, food becomes a delicious, nurturing, sensual experience. Why deprive ourselves of this pleasure? Joy does not come from settling for low-fat fromage frais with sugar-free jam. Joy comes from a freshly baked apricot cheesecake. Happiness isn't in that third packet of Maltesers bought furtively at the corner shop. Happiness is eating Maltesers really, really slowly, sucking the chocolate off each one before crunching the inside. Pleasure isn't about stashing away enough points to qualify for a serving of frozen yoghurt. Pleasure is going to Häagen-Dazs for dinner and tasting every flavour available. It's not fun weighing ourselves every morning only to discover we are still pounds away from that ever elusive target weight. Fun is using the scales to weigh your luggage before a low-cost trip to the beach!

The diet mentality, which requires us to measure and count every aspect of our lives, from grams of fat to calories burned, forces us into a rigid existence that leaves little space for spontaneity and joy. Most women who come on our workshops associate dieting or being good with guilt. Guilt permeates every aspect of their relationship with food and their body, making it hard to enjoy anything.

Over and over again on workshops we hear how guilty women feel and how often they beat themselves up for not getting it right, doing it properly or sticking to a long list of 'shoulds' 'musts' and 'ought-tos'. The variety is mind-boggling and seemingly endless. Here are just a few examples that we have heard over the years . . . (the names are made up for obvious reasons but the examples aren't!):

Bella gets up in the morning and feels guilty because she can't get into most of the clothes in her wardrobe. It's about time she really knuckled down and took the diet seriously.

Betty feels guilty as she rushes to work gobbling down a muffin and skinny latte; she knows a good healthy breakfast would be so much better for her and they do say it's the most important meal of the day . . .

Belinda feels guilty at lunchtime because she had planned to go to the gym but her colleagues were trying out the new café down the road so she joined them instead. She feels guilty at tea break because she ate four chocolate digestives that she didn't even really want.

Becky feels guilty because after the morning rush, getting the kids ready and ferrying them to school and battling with the traffic, she puts her feet up with a cup of tea and polishes off half a bag of fun-sized Mars Bars which were meant for their packed lunches.

Beth feels guilty because she nibbles at peanuts all afternoon, sitting at the PC while she pretends to work on that complicated report she can't quite get to grips with.

Barbara feels guilty because she's been delving into the biscuit tin all afternoon, even though she's not hungry and doesn't even particularly fancy biscuits.

Brenda feels guilty because she went to the cinema last night after a lovely Chinese meal and still couldn't resist the popcorn.

Beverly feels guilty because she polished off all the children's left-over tea (fish fingers, peas and those yummy chocolate pots) and now she's sitting down to supper with her husband who hates eating alone, even though she's not in the slightest bit hungry.

Beatrice feels guilty because she spent all evening in front of the telly and has finished off a jumbo bag of tortilla chips.

Bianca feels guilty because she was invited out to dinner and had everything from starter to pudding, and she was supposed to be sticking to her diet.

Ditch the guilt

Guilt is so unhelpful. We feel bad about ourselves and then . . . we eat some more! Freedom from all that guilt is possibly the most liberating part of Beyond Chocolate. In fact, as far as most workshop participants are concerned it's even better than the weight loss. Knowing that we no longer have to berate ourselves for eating chocolate or having a second helping of cheesecake, that guilt is no more part of our vocabulary than diets or calories or points is so liberating. Learning how to ditch the guilt means that we can really truly enjoy food, any food, without that sinking feeling.

It's only when we give ourselves permission to eat the foods we really like when we are hungry for them that we can enjoy eating. It is only when we truly take the time to savour each mouthful that food can become pleasurable. It is only when we start talking back to those critical voices with which we accuse ourselves of everything from being fat and ugly to totally lacking in willpower that we can start to enjoy the body we are in. When we do these things, we replace guilt with enjoyment and fun.

Kay Stevens, from London, did an eight-week course in London

Before

❛ I used to eat "healthy" meals – vegetable stir-fries with tofu, salads for dinner, sandwiches on wholegrain bread with fruit for lunch. But I also nibbled just a little bit whenever I passed the fridge or the cupboard – a small slice of cheese, a couple of olives, a few cashew nuts. It was as though, if I didn't dirty any crockery, and rinsed the knife or spoon I'd used straight away, it didn't count. So I'd nibble for an hour or so then cook a "proper" meal – which I'd eat too, even though I wasn't really hungry for it. ❜

Now

❝ Since the Beyond Chocolate workshop, I take a special plate and make a platter of my favourite foods – olives, cubes of mature Cheddar, cherry tomatoes, cashew nuts. I arrange them nicely, pour myself a gin and tonic or a glass of wine, light a candle and put on some music, then sit down and enjoy. And that is my dinner. I no longer cook food I don't want just because I should; instead I eat what I want without guilt – and enjoy it ten times more! ❞

ACTION!

A good place to start:

Have some fun!

How can you bring the enjoyment and fun back into eating? Here are some ideas that participants came up with on our workshops:

Have a children's tea party . . . for the adults, with jelly and ice cream, Twiglets, Iced Gems, sausages on sticks, chocolate fingers, lemon squash and the rest.

Bake lots of fairy cakes and decorate each one with different-coloured icing, silver balls and hundreds-and-thousands for a party, instead of stocking up at M&S.

Go out for a meal to your local restaurant and try a dish you've never had. Do this until you've tried everything that tempts you on the menu and then try a new restaurant.

continued

Invite friends round for a themed meal; you could serve dinners from around the world or a meal where all the food is one colour.

Experiment with different foods – educate your palate. Go out and buy a fruit or vegetable you've never eaten before. Log on to the Internet to find a recipe if you're not sure what to do with it.

Eat a meal with your fingers only.

Invest in a good cookbook with basic recipes for all occasions. Delia Smith and Nigel Slater's books are classics and we love the mouth-watering photos in all of Nigella Lawson's cookbooks.

Eat a Bourbon biscuit (or a custard cream) by opening it up and licking all the chocolatey bit off first before eating the biscuit.

Make 'fish-pond jelly' with slices of clementine to look like the goldfish and pieces of angelica for the seaweed.

Have a chocolate blind-tasting – with everything from Cadbury's Dairy Milk to the very best dark chocolate.

Make a wicked dessert such as tiramisu or fresh-cream meringue decorated with cream and strawberries and have it because it's *not* your birthday.

Be your own chef! Copy the recipes you've seen them making on TV.

Have a candle-lit breakfast to brighten up a winter's morning and make it special.

REALITY CHECK

It's a pleasure

We've all heard that stress is unhealthy, so we can safely assume that pleasure is good for us. Food and eating can provide great pleasure, especially when we eat food we like. The main reason we prefer one food over another is because of its flavour. And flavour is actually made up of several sensations that we experience simultaneously: taste, smell and touch (temperature and texture). Flavour can change completely when even one of these sensations is diminished. The right atmosphere can also make a big difference. It's no coincidence that fast-food outlets are decked out with neon lighting and plastic seating – no one wants to linger over a burger, it's not about enjoyment and pleasure, it's about quick profits. Eating in a comfortable, inviting environment highlights flavours and therefore our enjoyment of them and we're all the healthier for it.

> **? DID YOU KNOW . . .**
>
> In *La Physiologie du Gout* (*The Physiology of Taste*), 1826, Brillat-Savarin said: 'Animals feed themselves, men eat: but only wise men know the art of eating.'
> Wise women too!

I taste the freedom when . . . I eat Nutella straight from the jar with my fingers.

Food for thought

- What feelings do you associate with food?
- How will you have fun with food?
- What foods do you really enjoy?

Tune in

Eat when you are hungry

Eat whatever you want

Put it on a plate, sit down and focus

Stop when you are satisfied

Enjoy

Own your body

Move!

Support yourself

Be your own guru

CHAPTER • 10

Mirror, mirror on the wall

Having a healthy relationship with food goes hand in hand with having a healthy relationship with your body. Starting to own the body you have *now* is the best way to ensure that you get the body you want.

Before

Whenever I looked in the mirror I would criticise myself from head to toe. There were very few parts of my body that I liked and I would beat myself up with nasty comments. I would have given anything to get rid of my disgustingly flabby arm wings, to chop off those revolting rolls of fat around my midriff and suck out all the fat from my lumpy thighs. Other people's scrutiny was even worse than looking in the mirror. I got so sick of hearing, 'What a shame, you have such a pretty face.' Even when the comments were flattering I didn't believe them. I felt enormous, as big as a house, whatever I weighed.

Going to the beach was excruciating, even in the shapeless

kaftan I hid under. I couldn't begin to contemplate wearing a bikini. To do that, I would have to look like one of the impossibly beautiful and toned women that populated the pages of the magazines I browsed through as I lay self-consciously on the sunbed.

I would go to parties and, instead of enjoying the company, the music, the food, I would spend most of my time checking out and comparing myself to other women in the room. If there were some who were fatter than me I felt better about myself – prettier, funnier. I would spend most of the evening thinking about my body, about how fat I was. I analysed the thin women with total precision: their bottoms, their thighs, their breasts, and automatically assumed that they were happy, successful and in control – all the things I wanted so badly for myself. Sometimes, I would end up going home because I was so ashamed. I felt so fat and disgusting that I didn't want to be around people. I wanted to be at home under the duvet, eating myself into oblivion and zapping through the 999 channels on my television.

I dreamed of waking up in the morning at my ideal weight, thin, miraculously toned and finally ready. Ready for what? Oh, everything: to look for a better job, to go to the swimming pool, to meet Mr Right, to sign up for that creative writing class, to eat really healthily, to wax – even in winter. In the meantime, though, I hated my body and tortured it with endless attempts at weight loss. Some of them even worked for a while but, somehow, I never felt thin enough to make those changes.

Now

I look in the mirror and marvel at my body. I love my curves and even my lumps and bumps, affectionately known as 'squidgy bits'. I have the sumptuous body of a 30-something woman who has a story to tell. When I look at women I see how beautiful they are; all the women who come to our workshops, desperate to change, are beautiful already. I look after my body and it looks after me. As a thank you to my legs for holding me up all day and helping me sprint up that hill, I treat them to a lavender foot soak. I wear clothes that I like and that really fit me, no more kaftans. Oh, and I wax – even in January.

What happened?

I attended a women's workshop in which we were set some fascinating homework. To spend 20 minutes looking at ourselves naked in the mirror, as if we were seeing the first woman in the world, so no comparisons, judgements or criticisms were possible, as there was no defining standard. As I stood there I noticed how beautiful my eyes were, how smooth my skin was, how voluptuous my breasts were and marvelled at my elegant and dainty feet.

Doing this exercise highlighted how I constantly criticised my body and that I avoided looking at myself in the mirror too closely. It became obvious that changing my approach to weight loss went hand in hand with changing my relationship with my body.

I began to accept my body as it was, rather than waiting for that ever-elusive thinness. It's what I had, for better, for worse, I might as well make friends with it. I painted my toenails letter-box red and loved the way they peeped through the bubbles in the bath, I made time for beauty days, not just fancy expensive ones at the spa, but an evening in my bathroom with good music, candles and lots of lovely creams and potions. I bought myself a comfortable swimming costume and went to the local pool.

I still had days when I reverted to 'fat mode', when all I could hear were the critical and nasty comments I threw at myself. That's when I started to talk back and to take control. I wasn't going to let that nasty little gremlin on my shoulder put me down. Every time it spouted its poison I cut it off with the same retort 'If you don't have anything helpful to say, SHUT UP!' End of conversation. It took time; the gremlin was loud and persistent, but the more I stood up to it the quieter it got and the better I felt about myself.

Whenever I compared myself to other women I would find ways to appreciate them instead of envying their imagined happiness and perfection. I reminded myself that these were just ordinary women, who probably had the same doubts and worries as me, and had bad-hair days – the size and shape of their body didn't come into it.

What it boils down to

We have grown up in a culture that celebrates women who are thin, toned, have a healthy 'glow' and wear fashionable clothes. The images that surround us in the media, be it film, magazines, television or billboards, overwhelmingly send out the message that a successful, happy woman is beautiful, stylish and, above all, thin. These are powerful, insidious images and messages that many of us make into the rules by which we live our lives. We dedicate ourselves to achieving these goals of beauty and thinness in order, we hope, to be successful and happy.

Being thin and being happy are not synonymous

Many of us have been thin and unhappy. We have been thin and 'unsuccessful'; we have been thin and out of control.

Success, happiness, stability – none of these can be achieved through a body size – if only it were that simple. The size of your body does not determine the size of your life. It never has and never will. And yet many of us live as though the two are dependent on each other. True confidence and self-esteem do not come from anything as ephemeral as our appearance. Confidence and self-esteem come from learning to like ourselves and love ourselves whatever packaging we come in.

Fitness not thinness

We live in an increasingly fat-phobic society in which we are constantly told that losing weight will make us more beautiful and that it is the answer to almost all our health problems. However, cutting-edge, independent studies are consistently showing that a person's weight is not necessarily linked with their health. A slim couch potato is in no way healthier than an active 'overweight' person. It's not the size of our body that determines how healthy we are it's our level of fitness, and it's perfectly possible to be fit and 'overweight'. In fact yo-yo dieting, which leads to repeatedly losing and then gaining weight, is *more* dangerous for our health than weight gain. There are several fascinating books on this subject written by scientists and researchers who explain it infinitely better than we can: *The Obesity Myth* by Paul Campos and *Big Fat Lies* by Glenn Gaesser (see Further reading, page 242).

People whose weight has fluctuated up and down are more likely to have health problems than overweight people whose weight remains stable or who put on more weight. So when we are told that the main reason we need to lose weight is to be healthy, we need to think again.

We can't expect to change something we refuse to own

Motivation for change does not come from reminding ourselves daily that we are unattractive and unlovable, and by rejecting our bodies. Beating ourselves up like punchbags is demoralising, demeaning and self-defeating. The way we talk to and about ourselves can have an enormous impact on the way we feel about ourselves. By criticising and judging our bodies, and constantly making the kind of remarks that we would never say to our friends or loved ones, we bash our self-esteem, which often leads to more eating. Real, lasting change (including weight loss) comes from awareness of who we are and accepting ourselves just as we are, right now. We can start to live our lives *now*, whatever we weigh.

Caroline McAdam, from London, came on a weekend workshop in London

Before

❝ Beyond Chocolate has changed my life. When I was first introduced to the approach I was appalled! I thought, "There's no way this can possibly work! If I fill my kitchen with my favourite food, I'll give into temptation immediately and never stop." I regarded myself as being out of control around food and while I loved cooking I felt it was something that I should avoid as far as possible. For me, becoming thin was all that mattered. Everything would be all right then. My experience of losing weight was of self-denial and misery followed by cravings and failure, but I was so desperate to succeed, I told myself that it was my weakness that was letting me down, which of course made me feel all the more miserable. The idea that no food was "bad" or "forbidden" seemed like a recipe for disaster. How could I possibly lose weight like this?

I want to laugh now remembering that my focus, to the exclusion of everything else, was on losing weight. I saw myself and my value as a person in terms of my size and weight – the less I weighed, the more acceptable I was. In the previous year I'd lost and quickly regained three stone and felt a complete failure. Angry, worthless and hopeless. ⦆

Now

⦅ Applying the Beyond Chocolate principles has been a revelation. For the first time in my life I am eating and enjoying the food I really want without guilt. I have quickly discovered how powerful and liberating this is and how not feeling guilty, not telling myself that what I am eating is bad, means that I have broken the vicious circle of self-criticism and eating for comfort, and that I am not out of control at all. I have lost weight and it has stayed off. I've gradually come to see the extent to which I used food as an emotional support and that at the heart of this lay my lack of self-confidence and need over reassurance and comfort.

I am very clear now that body size has little to do with self-confidence. Self-confidence comes from self-knowledge and self-awareness and while I would like to lose more weight I know that the key to my happiness and contentment lies in working on those difficult feelings I used food to alleviate. I have realised how incredibly critical I was towards myself and how damaging this was. I have learned the positive effects of being compassionate towards myself and I am so much happier as a result. ⦆

A smaller size has its benefits: it is easier to buy clothes, it can make movement less of an effort and it may or may not be beneficial for our health[1]. Full stop.

I asked a past participant at a support session a few weeks ago how her life has changed now that she has a much healthier relationship with food and that she feels good about her body. She mentioned feeling free and more confident, she talked about the liberation of never having to diet and eating the food she likes, she told me about the delight of buying clothes that she feels good in and she explained that she has taken some of the Beyond Chocolate principles and applied them to other areas in her life. When another participant asked her if all this was because she had finally lost weight, she laughed. 'You know it isn't,' she said, 'it has nothing to do with the size of my body.'

What it boils down to is this: if we spend our lives focusing on our body size, rejecting the body we have and wishing it were different, dreaming of the day when, slim and perfect, our life will finally start, then we spend our whole life waiting and we miss the chance to live our lives fully now.

J.H., from Kingston, did the multimedia course

6 I can't describe the change I feel. I weighed myself as I know I have lost some weight and think I've lost about 11lbs although I'm not precisely sure of the starting weight – I feel fitter, healthier, cleaner inside and mentally so much more in control and forward looking. And when I weighed myself it was nice but not the big deal it used to be. 9

Victoria, from London, came on a weekend workshop in London

Before

6 I would weigh myself each morning without fail while praying, with no clothes on, after going to the loo and before breakfast. The number on the scales would decide my mood for

the whole day. If the number was lower than I expected I would have a 'pig-out day'. I figured that I had a few pounds to play around with. If the number was higher than I expected I would be devastated and the day would be ruined, no matter what. 〕

Now

〔 I have thrown my scales in a skip. I wake up each morning and sometimes I feel fantastic, sometimes pretty ordinary. I now realise that "that's life" with all its ups and downs. I now realise that fat days are not about the fat; if you dig a little deeper you can figure out what's really going on inside you. 〕

ACTION!

A good place to start:

Get to know your body.
Spend some time *really* looking at yourself naked in a full-length mirror, make it just a few minutes a couple of times a week. Start by focusing on your face or your legs or a part of you that you like. Aim to see yourself without judgement or criticism; just notice what you see, keep to the facts and avoid comparisons. If the idea of doing that freaks you out, start small: do it with your clothes on and spend a few minutes every day naked, in the privacy of your bathroom. Get to know your body, make friends with it.

Body language

Think of a critical, judgemental comment that you have made to your body or about your body in the last 24 hours or something that you know you often say; for example, 'I've got such a fat arse' (sometimes it's more subtle than that). Tune in to the thoughts that go through your head and listen to what you tell yourself about your body. Are you nasty and critical (for example, 'Those flabby arm wings are disgusting, I can't wear a sleeveless top looking like that'), or miserable and self-pitying (for example, 'Oh it's so unfair, why have I got so much horrid cellulite on my thighs'). Whether you beat yourself up or put yourself down, experiment with finding a way to silence that gremlin – whatever works for you. It could be telling it to shut up, or something along those lines. If you can't think of anything to say that works for you that's fine. Stick to noticing how you criticise yourself. Just acknowledging that you do this can start to make all the difference.

Self-defence

Don't let other people say negative things about your body either. Instead of quietly putting up with it or aggressively attacking them, find out what happens when you ask them the following question: 'And you're saying that because . . .?' Most of the time they won't know what to say and if they think about it, even for a minute, they're unlikely to do it again.

Dear body

Write a letter to your body. Start your letter off with: Dear Body. Tell it exactly how you feel about it. Be as spontaneous and honest as you can.

When you have finished, start another letter and write Dear [add your name]. Now give your body a chance to reply. With your non-dominant hand write a reply from your body to yourself (if you're right handed that means using your left hand, and vice versa – writing with your other hand accesses a different part of the brain).

Allow yourself to be surprised by what you write. Almost all of the participants on our workshops say that this is a very powerful and moving exercise.

It's good to talk

Have a conversation with your fat. Write it down if you like. If you don't feel fat, talk to the part of you that has an issue with food or body image.

Example:

Me: 'Hello Fat. Are you there?'
Fat: 'Where else would I be?'
Me: 'Oh God! I wish you'd just disappear.'
Fat: 'Well I never asked to be here, I'm not the one who ate a whole tub of Ben & Jerry's last night.'
And so on.
Make your conversation as long as you like.

Have some aahh time

We all deserve to look after ourselves, whatever our size. Make time to look after your body. It could be moving more (see Chapter 12) or having beauty or relaxing treatments such as letting someone massage away the cares of day. Put your feet in a lavender foot soak and do *nothing* for five minutes. The more you do these things the better you will like yourself and the less you'll turn to food. A beauty day doesn't have to be at the spa. Treat your body to a home-made beauty session. Put on some good music and get down to business. Wax, pluck, shave, knead, exfoliate, massage, moisturise, cleanse, steam, sponge, smooth and brush.

Ditch the scales

Why let a little black number dictate your mood and self-esteem every day? Especially when those numbers are mean-ingless. So ditch the scales or keep them just to make sure you won't have to pay excess luggage fees when you next fly off on holiday.

Flatter yourself

Pick four of the words below that describe your body. On a piece of card, write: 'I am . . .' followed by the four words and place it somewhere you can see it.

Voluptuous	Radiant	Sexy	Sensual	Curvaceous
Rounded	Shapely	Smooth	Strong	Agile
Supple	Soft	Silky	Womanly	Feminine
Firm	Graceful	Elegant	Healthy	Fit
Dynamic	Tanned	Glowing	Fulsome	Shining
Peaches and cream	English rose	Vibrant	Stylish	Smart

REALITY CHECK

The truth about bathroom scales

Is your mood dictated by the little number that appears between your feet every morning? Do you rejoice when the scales tell you that you have lost a pound, and do you plunge into despair when it seems you have put two on overnight? Well, think again because there are many factors that influence the numbers on the scales. Daily weight fluctuations are normal, they are not indicators of success or failure. Once you understand how these mechanisms work, you can free yourself from the daily battle with the bathroom scales.

Normal fluctuations in the body's water content can hugely influence body weight. Two factors that affect water retention are water consumption and salt intake. Bizarrely, the less you drink, the more your body will hang on to water supplies. Salt intake can also play a big role in water retention. The more highly processed a food is, the more likely it is to have a high sodium (salt) content. Therefore, if you are dehydrated, or have eaten foods containing a lot of salt, you are likely to weigh more.

Women are also likely to fluctuate in weight according to menstrual cycles. It is normal to weigh more prior to menstruation.

Another factor that can influence your weight is glycogen storage. Think of glycogen as the body's fuel. It is made up of carbohydrates and water and can weigh up to 2.25kg (5lb). As you use the fuel up during the day, and the reserves shrink, you will get increasingly hungry, and when you eat you will replenish your body's energy reserve. It's normal to experience glycogen and water weight shifts of up to 1kg (2lb) per day even with no changes in your calorie intake or activity level. These fluctuations have nothing to do with fat loss.

Otherwise rational people also tend to forget about the actual weight of the food they eat. The 1.8kg (4lb) that you gain the morning after a huge dinner is not fat. It's the actual weight of everything you've had to eat and drink. The added weight of the meal will be gone several hours later when you have finished digesting it.

Also, weight gain doesn't necessarily mean fat gain. Actually, to store the above dinner as 2.25kg (5lb) of fat, it would have to contain a whopping 17,500 calories. That would mean eating a meal made up of:

20 vol-au-vents
20 cocktail sausages
6 glasses of champagne
2 × 30cm (12in) pepperoni pizzas
half a leg of roast lamb
2 helpings of mashed potatoes
4 helpings of broccoli
a whole family-sized dish of cauliflower cheese
450g (1lb) of Cheddar cheese and a packet of crackers
2 Caesar salads
3 bottles of beer
an entire apple pie with a giant tub of vanilla ice cream
4 cappuccino coffees
1 box of 40 After Eight mints

Is this humanly possible? So when the scales go up by 1.4g or 1.8kg (3lb or 4lb) overnight, it's likely to be water, glycogen, and the weight of your dinner.

This brings us to the scales' sneakiest attribute: they don't just weigh fat. They weigh muscle, bone, water, internal organs and all. When you lose 'weight' that doesn't necessarily mean that you have lost fat. In fact, the scales have no way of telling you what you've lost (or gained). The problem with the scales is that they don't differentiate between any of these.

? DID YOU KNOW . . .

Beauty mags give women the blues. In a study[2] on the influence of fashion magazines on body-image satisfaction, researchers discovered that after only 13 minutes, women who had been given fashion magazines to read reported more frequently:

- Feeling very frustrated about their weight.

- Thinking about dieting.

- Exercising only to lose weight.

- Weighing themselves more than once a week.

- Feeling guilty while and after eating.

- Being preoccupied with the desire to be thinner.

- Being afraid of getting fat.

So be more selective about what you read; you don't have to go all serious, treat yourself to some "feel-good" chick lit where the heroine lives happily ever after.

I taste the freedom when . . . I dance naked around my living room.

Food for thought

◉ How do you feel when you look in the mirror?

◉ What are you putting off until you have lost weight?

◉ How often do you compare yourself to other women? How do you feel when you do it?

◉ What kind of things does your gremlin say?

CHAPTER 11

Every item in my wardrobe fits just right

Wearing clothes that we like, that feel comfortable and that fit, whatever our size, can make an enormous difference to how confident we feel in our bodies. Whatever your budget, you can enjoy looking great and start feeling good about your body right now.

Before

My weight went up and down like a yo-yo. I had my thin clothes and my fat clothes, and I never threw any away. When I was feeling fat, I would try on my thin jeans, just to see if I could squeeze into them. They were white Levis, which I had been slim enough to wear for about six weeks one summer, and every day I dreamed of being thin enough to fit into them again. I hated my poor body more every time. I put off buying beautiful clothes until I was thin, and I squeezed myself into clothes that were too small. When I did go shopping, I bought big and baggy although I was dying to wear fitted and stylish but they either didn't come in my size or I didn't have the guts to wear them.

Every day when I opened the wardrobe door to get dressed I would be faced with piles of T-shirts two sizes too small, trousers that wouldn't get past my thighs and dresses that wouldn't do up. These clothes were a constant reminder that I was too big, that my body was letting me down, that it really was high time to summon up the willpower to be 'good' and get a grip. And every day I had a good reason to tell myself how fat I was, and inevitably I would feel bad about myself and my body.

I bought more clothes in larger sizes to fit me (after all, I needed *something* to wear to work) but avoided spending too much because I was definitely planning to lose weight and it would be such a waste to buy expensive clothes that would sit there unworn when I was slim (which I promised myself would be soon).

Shopping was so depressing and disappointing. I told myself that black and grey were elegant and flattering. I donned floaty, shadowy numbers that covered me up and avoided defining my shape. And when I did lose weight, I kept my fat clothes at the back of the wardrobe, just in case.

Now

My weight fluctuates little. I don't keep clothes in my wardrobe that I don't like or that don't fit. I have far fewer clothes than I used to but I know that every single item fits and feels good. Getting dressed in the morning is fine, except when I can't find a top to wear because they are all in the ironing pile. Every season I have a 'sort out' and give any unwanted items to friends or to a charity shop. When I go shopping I still buy quite a lot of black and grey, but I also treat myself to lovely bright pink fitted tops, sparkly belts and bikinis in the summer. I even splash out on lacy, sexy underwear, just for myself. I feel confident in my clothes and I really love the way I look.

What happened?

When I started paying more attention to my body, I realised how depressing and punishing my wardrobe was. One afternoon I decided to have a good old sort out. I emptied my wardrobe and chest of drawers and I sat on my bedroom floor surrounded by every item of clothing I possessed. I looked at each one in turn and decided whether I liked it or not and tried it on to see if it fitted. I had a huge black bin bag destined for Oxfam, for the clothes that I knew I would never wear again, even if I could fit into them. I put all my favourites in a suitcase and stored it in the loft, I couldn't bring myself to give them away just yet but I knew that seeing them every single day was neither encouraging nor motivating. All they did was to remind me of what a failure I was. I made another pile of items that I had once loved but knew I'd never wear again; these were all quite expensive and good quality, so I decided to give them to friends and family who I knew would really appreciate them.

Then I went out and bought myself a few things that I really liked, that fitted me well and that I felt good in. I didn't quite have the courage to go for bold, fitted tops but I found a really nice linen shirt and a couple of funky T-shirts that were certainly more flattering than the items I had just evacuated. And I invested in a really good pair of jeans that were cut to fit me just right – I felt really good in them.

What it boils down to

Wear clothes that you like and feel good in. Having thin clothes and fat clothes hanging in our wardrobes is telling ourselves every day that we need to lose weight. We might as well have a poster hanging there saying YOU ARE A FAIL-URE! Our thin clothes are a reminder of all the times we lost the weight and put it all back on again and the fat clothes tell us not to believe in ourselves because, diet or no diet, we'll be back into them before long.

It's not only about the size, if we don't feel comfortable in our clothes and we don't like the way we look it's bound to dam-age our self-esteem and it certainly doesn't motivate us. Bonnie, one of our more adventurous participants, kept a blog. One day her entry was all about how uncomfortable she felt in her clothes: 'I've realised that I'm wearing trousers that are much too tight. The waistband digs into my stomach and so I'm con-stantly thinking about how fat I am. It's really depressing. I've decided to go out and buy myself a few things that fit properly.'

ACTION!

A good place to start:

Spring clean!
Get some large bin bags, suitcases and boxes. Go through every item in your wardrobe and ask yourself these questions: does it fit? Do I really like it? Have I worn it this year? If the answer to any of them is no then put it in the Oxfam pile, or the loft pile, or the give-to-friends pile.

continued

Make sure that all the items you put back in your wardrobe fit just right. They might not all be your favourites, there may be some you need to keep even though you are not madly keen on them, we can't all afford a new wardrobe just like that. Slowly but surely you can replace them with ones you really like.

If your budget allows, buy yourself a few new things that you feel good in. Do some research, find out which shops and designers cater to your particular body shape and size in a style that you like. There's so much out there.

Get your friends to do it, too, and have a girls' night in where everyone brings a bagful – you'll be surprised at how well this can work. The jeans your best friend hates so much could be perfect for you.

At the very least buy yourself one item that you really like and that makes you feel good. It could be anything, from that designer coat you've always wanted to a pair of funky tights. What would it be for you?

Make it special, give it some thought: what shops would you like to go to? Would you rather go alone or with a friend? Make whatever arrangements you need to ensure that you have a good time.

REALITY CHECK . . .

What's in a dress size?

According to the BCIA (British Clothing Industry & Association), each retailer is making clothes to fit a target market, so a retailer for 16 to 24 year olds is going to have a different combination of sizes from the retailer aiming for the over forties. In other words, a size 14 skirt in Topshop may be the same size as a size 10 skirt in Marks & Spencer. Sizing is totally arbitrary and varies from shop to shop.

Some retailers label their clothes with smaller sizes to make us feel good; this is called 'vanity sizing' – they hope that we will buy the trousers just because we feel good that they are a size smaller than the last ones we bought. Then we can kid ourselves that the diet's working. The dress size you wear bears almost no relation to the size of your body!

And sizes are getting smaller, size 6 has only recently made an appearance on the high street. As we career towards 0 (which already exists in the US) it begs the question: is being 0, nothing, invisible, the ideal we are aiming for?

Most research shows that the average British woman is a size 16. The sad truth is that many of the more fashionable high-street shops never display size 16 clothes on the shop floor, or when they do, there are so few that, surprise, surprise, they go as soon as they hit the rail.

? DID YOU KNOW . . .

Carrie Otis, a top fashion model, confessed: 'My diet was really starvation, I am not really naturally that thin, so I had to go through everything from using drugs to diet pills to laxatives to fasting. Those were my main ways of controlling my weight.' The average model weighs 23 per cent less than the average English woman. No wonder Carrie had to starve to fit into the clothes that she modelled and that we would all love to wear.

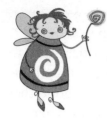

*I taste the freedom when . . . I
wear a fitted pink T-shirt
and feel fab.*

Food for thought

◉ How do you feel about the clothes in your wardrobe?

◉ What will you do with the clothes you don't want or need?

◉ What one item of clothing can you go out and buy yourself now?

Tune in

Eat when you are hungry

Eat whatever you want

Put it on a plate, sit down and focus

Stop when you are satisfied

Enjoy

Own your body

Move!

Support yourself

Be your own guru

CHAPTER 12

Work it out

Moving our bodies is vital for health and fitness, whatever our size. It doesn't have to be hard work, time-consuming or expensive. Finding enjoyable, realistic ways to stay in shape is beneficial for our overall health and is the indispensable companion to a healthy relationship with food for permanent, sustainable weight loss.

Before

Exercise was something I dreaded. It was always part of a weight-loss scheme. I would start a new diet – and a new exercise plan at the same time. The end objective of any physical activity was to tone muscle and lose fat. When I wasn't on a diet, exercise was a way of making up for 'pigging out' or an attempt to shift some weight before the summer holidays and the dreaded bikini season. The various self-inflicted regimes of torture I set up for myself included joining an endless list of gyms, employing a personal trainer, signing up for aerobics, yoga, step, swearing to myself that I would swim 25 lengths three times a week, anything that promised me a body like the one I dreamed of: trim, toned and tanned.

My experience of exercise was awful and usually ended up in dismal failure. I would sign up for whatever class I had chosen with the best of intentions. After an initial period of 'being good', I would start to skip classes, finding perfect excuses not to go. When I did drag myself to whichever activity I'd chosen that month, I usually didn't even enjoy it, enduring boredom, pain and, worst of all, wet clammy hair on a cold winter's evening after a mind-numbing session in a bath of chlorine. What started out as a three-times-a-week routine slowly became twice a week, then once, then only occasionally – always fuelled by guilt.

At this stage I would usually come to the conclusion that there was no point in going if I wasn't going to do it 'properly' and I would give up altogether, promising myself that I would start again next Monday, next month, next year . . . exactly the way I approached diets. The reality is that I only did it because I thought it would help me achieve the perfect body, which it never did.

Now

I have completely changed the way I think about exercise and my body. Not only is a slim, toned body no longer something I yearn for ten times a day, I know that using my body, moving and stretching my muscles, filling my lungs and working my heart are about being fit and healthy not slim and attractive. Today I *move* because I derive pleasure from using my body in ways that work for me. I have banished the words 'should' or 'must' from my vocabulary.

I no longer think that unless I am following a routine and

doing exercise on a regular basis then it's not worth doing. I tune into my body and find out what type of movement fits for me on any given day. Sometimes I do some simple yoga stretches in my living room, or I drop into a local class, other times I head down to the pool. I went to see an osteopath who suggested a few movements that I could do to improve my posture and help with my backache. They take less than 20 minutes and I like doing them. I even learned to run. I say learned because I was absolutely sure that I couldn't do it. I thought it was just part of my make up – I was the type of woman who can't run. So I asked a friend who runs for pleasure how she does it and she explained. I tried it out for myself and I could hardly believe the sheer pleasure of being able to run for 25 minutes non-stop and still not feel out of breath. Any attempt I had ever made before ended in a stitch and heavy panting after two minutes – at best. Movement has become an important, enjoyable part of my life, which I look forward to rather than enduring.

What happened?

As I started to change my approach to weight loss and develop a new relationship with my body, I changed the way I thought about exercise. I realised that 'exercise' did not necessarily mean slogging it out at the gym three times a week or following a military-type regime that I didn't enjoy and gave me no flexibility. Like my hunger, my appetite for movement varied according to the time of the year, the time of the month – and even the time of day. As long as I approached exercise in the same way I had approached dieting – with that all-or-nothing mentality – I would continue to set myself rules that I couldn't stick to.

I became curious as to what type of exercise I enjoyed and

what really didn't work for me. I began to experiment with different types that didn't involve signing up to a gym or to a class which I would feel obliged to go to (and then feel like a failure if I didn't). Because I didn't feel that I *had* to go, it was then a question of choice. I understood that, for me, variation was fundamental. A brisk walk round the park one morning, a drop-in yoga session and a swim in the sea if it was summer, or a dance around my living room in winter, were great ways of moving my body which I really enjoyed. It didn't feel like a duty any more. The realisation that I could have fun and enjoy moving my body and that I could do this when and where I fancied – and still classify it as exercise, made all the difference.

What it boils down to

Moving our bodies is vital for our health but too often we see exercise exclusively as a means to weight loss. Learning to dissociate exercise from weight loss is the key, whatever your size. If we can see beyond the need to have an exercise regime with the sole aim of losing weight and toning muscle, we stand some chance of finding ways of looking after our health and maintaining an appropriate level of fitness that is not only good for us but also satisfying.

Movement is social, playful and pleasurable; it's for enjoyment and improved quality of life and better health, not for calorie burning and weight loss. Take the focus away from what your body looks like, to what your body can do for you. On our Summer Retreat we offer yoga on the terrace every morning. Everybody loves it, from the experienced yogis to the absolute beginners. We were really lucky to come across the right teacher; Gareth (see page 218) has the same approach to yoga as Beyond Chocolate has to food. Slowly does it, do what you can – the aim is to tune in and enjoy.

The reason we need 'to exercise' at all is because as humans we were not designed to sit staring at a screen for eight hours a day. We are programmed to have physically active lifestyles: hunting, running, walking, climbing, carrying, fetching, digging, hoeing, and so on. As one participant in a workshop said, 'That makes sense, if I was getting up every morning and going to work in the fields, I wouldn't need to join the gym!'

The irony is, when movement has its rightful place in our lives, when we do it regularly and enjoy it, when we use our body with energy and delight we will be burning fat, too. It's a consequence, not the goal. The minute we focus on it as a means to weight loss alone, we will find ways to sabotage ourselves just like we sabotaged the diets.

Start now

It is so easy to put off using our bodies until we find the right time and the right activity. We can always find a reason why today is not a good day, this week is not a good week. Nike has the perfect motto: whatever you can do now, JUST DO IT!

Cathie Wilson, from Herefordshire, did a weekend workshop in Gloucestershire and the multimedia course

❝ I let myself join a *private* gym so that I can exercise in a kind environment, and I can go at any time that suits me, so if my schedule has to change, so can my exercise. I've let myself rediscover dance; my Christmas present was a music player and I sometimes put on the loudest CD I can find and spend up to an hour just dancing. Even though I couldn't exercise for a month when I put out a disc and then put on a few pounds, I didn't mind, I was just glad to be back on my feet. ❞

ACTION!

A good place to start:

Find out what you like doing.

Remember what filled you with glee when you were a child – what made your heart beat faster and brought a flush to your cheeks? Stomping through puddles, kicking up the autumn leaves, climbing a tree, riding your bike at breakneck speed, playing rounders with your friends in the park, spinning round and round, faster and faster until you felt dizzy? Find out what kind of activity you will really enjoy now. It doesn't have to be about slogging it at the gym. There are so many different ways to move and exercise our bodies. And it can be fun.

Once you have discovered an activity or several that you like, the key is to begin.

To stick with it, you have to find something you find acceptable at the very least, so experiment. There are so many different ways you can move your body that if you try out different options you will find something that works for you. If moving is not your thing, you may not grow to love it, but you will look forward to the endorphin release you get when you do it.

Start slowly and give yourself a chance. **Do not** make a plan to spend 30 minutes three times a week doing whatever movement it is you have discovered. Having improbable goals sets us up for failure. If you have not been moving much at all, planning to start a new regime three times a week is unrealistic and unhelpful. You don't have to have a punishing schedule or dedicate hours to

continued

wake up your muscles and activate your body. Even ten minutes each day can make a difference. It's a good start.

Aim to do a little and take it one day at a time. If you are the kind of person who likes the discipline of making an appointment in your diary, write it in one day at a time. If it becomes a duty or a chore, you will stop enjoying it and then stop doing it.

Afterwards notice how you feel – if you feel good, happier, healthier, more comfortable in your skin, then remind yourself of these feelings if you come up with resistance when you next plan to do it.

Tune in

Take a moment to tune in before, during and after moving your body.

Focus on the physical sensations: how does your body feel? What's aching? What feels good? What's stretched? What's relaxed?

How do you feel? Elated, exhausted, relaxed, invigorated?

Do you have any thoughts? If it wasn't great how could you improve it? If it was just right, when do you want to do it again?

Step by step

Once you start don't force yourself to make a commitment for the rest of your life. If you enjoy it, you may well want to do it for many years, but for now take one day at a time. When you have done an activity and enjoyed it once, commit to doing it again, one step at a time, one day at a time.

A problem shared is a problem halved

If it's a challenge to motivate yourself to go out for a walk or to the pool for a swim, how about finding a partner to go with you on a regular basis? Maybe you have a colleague at work who would like to use their lunch hour in this way. Or a neighbour who could walk to the park with you before work or in the evening. If you are not sure about asking people, how about posting a note through your neighbours' doors saying that you are looking for a walking partner. You could put up a notice at work or send an email. Having company can be a great way to help you keep committed, and can make it even more enjoyable.

Make it part of your schedule

Making time for movement is often one of the biggest obstacles to actually doing any. We lead such busy lives that we might relegate it to the bottom of the list. To help you make time for yourself so that you can use your body in a way you enjoy, make an appointment in your diary. Each week allow the time you would like to spend walking, dancing, playing tennis or whatever it is you want to do, and write it in ink. Treat this appointment with the same level of respect and commitment that you would another appointment, even if it's only ten minutes. It's as important as any business or social engagement, so make it a priority.

REALITY CHECK

Thin or fit?

There is a widely held assumption that overweight people are unhealthy and unfit and that slim people are the opposite. The fact is that neither is true.

In a study,[1] which tracked the relationship between the weight, fitness levels and health of more than 70,000 people over 20 years, statistics show that body mass appears to have no relevance to health whatsoever. Both the 'obese' and the 'moderately overweight' (whatever that means) who engage in at least moderate levels of physical activity have around half the mortality rate of sedentary people who maintain supposedly ideal body weights. Health and mortality rates were identical for all active people, regardless of their body size. The key to good health is movement, not weight loss.

 DID YOU KNOW . . .

A study[2] has found that improving your fitness levels by the equivalent of going for a brisk 30-minute walk four or five times a week reduces mortality rates by 50 per cent[3].

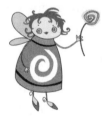 *I taste the freedom when . . . I walk because I can.*

Food for thought

Think of:

- One type of exercise/or movement you know you enjoy.

- One you do or have done but don't enjoy.

- One you have always wanted to try.

- One you do now, or could do, but don't consider to be exercise.

Tune in

Eat when you are hungry

Eat whatever you want

Put it on a plate, sit down and focus

Stop when you are satisfied

Enjoy

Own your body

Move!

Support yourself

Be your own guru

CHAPTER 13

Asking for help, not a second helping

We don't need to do everything on our own. Asking for help takes courage and strength and is not a sign of weakness. One of the main reasons we created Beyond Chocolate was to create the support that we wished we had for ourselves. Reach out, look around, and ask.

Before

I never asked for help, not from friends, family or anyone else. Partly because I was very proud and didn't like to admit that I needed it and partly because I was used to being seen as the strong one, the woman who could cope with anything. I juggled work and family commitments, I worked hard and played hard and was a relentlessly 'can do' kind of person. I came from a family where 'help' was for serious problems and I didn't see myself as having a serious problem. Being overweight and failing at diets hardly qualified as serious.

Professional help was totally out of the question. I didn't have a clue who to turn to anyway, and besides, I just needed to find the willpower to get on with it and stick to a plan. I could always moan to my girlfriends about how tough it was and how the latest diet hadn't worked – again – although I never really talked about the bingeing and the secret eating, when I was alone and miserable; I felt far too ashamed to actually admit that to anyone. Even though I knew I couldn't possibly be the only woman to stuff my sorrows down with yet another bowl of Crunchy Nut Corn Flakes, it felt like I was quite alone. None of my women friends had ever confessed to such depths, and I wasn't about to be the first. Food was always there when I needed support: readily available, no judgements, no expectations. Just an ever-present ally. And I paid the price as I piled on the pounds and felt even more miserable and out of control.

Now

My sister and I support each other and together we offer support to many women. I set aside ten minutes every morning to sit quietly, gather my thoughts, pick an angel card (see The Chocolate Fairy's favourite resources) and prepare for the day. I write in my journal regularly. I see a psychotherapist once a month and, as a therapist, I am in professional supervision (I am in a fortnightly supervision group with other therapists and an experienced supervisor) to support all the work that I do with Beyond Chocolate. I have surrounded myself with friends who understand and respect the choices I make, even if they do not always share them. I know I can turn to them for support at any time. Today I am much more likely to reach for the phone than for a bar of chocolate. I know that asking for help is a sign of my courage and self-respect. I trust in my ability to support myself and in my willingness to ask for help when I need it.

What happened?

A friend of mine went on a women's personal development weekend, and came back with a twinkle in her eye. She joined a women's group and seemed to relish the support and acceptance she received. I wanted some of that for myself and so I signed up; although a little sceptical and doubtful, I was hopeful. That weekend opened a door to a whole host of possibilities. I realised that I needed support and that my problem wasn't quite as simple as getting a grip and doing a diet properly, so I started to see a therapist. I also joined a monthly women's group, made time for myself, read inspiring books, and exchanged supportive emails and phone conversations with my sister and close friends. I found a whole host of ways to ensure that I did not feel alone with my struggle, and the more support I had, the less I felt the need to fill the void with food. I joined forces with my sister and we created Beyond Chocolate.

When we started we were very clear that we did not want to set up a system that would hook women in forever and keep them coming back for more. We wanted Beyond Chocolate to be an alternative to dieting, and to the dieting industry and its mechanisms. So for the first year, women would come on a workshop – end of story.

After a while we found that many women were asking for some form of ongoing support. So we provided it. Having a group of women who all know what you know and talk the same language is empowering and motivating. It's always good to know you're not alone.

What it boils down to

As women we are so good at supporting everyone around us that we forget that we, too, need support. We are caring mothers, loving partners, attentive daughters, sympathetic friends, loyal sisters and tireless colleagues. We are constantly under pressure, overwhelmed and overstimulated by demands at home and at work. We expect ourselves to be superwomen and everyone else does, too. No wonder we get stressed out, anxious and depressed. For many women, this translates into having an unhealthy relationship with food and their bodies. The only way we know to give ourselves a break or a treat is to eat something nice.

Once we have the tools and the practical solutions to transform our approach to weight loss, getting support makes it so much easier to keep ourselves motivated, encouraged and focused on transforming our relationship with food.

When we stop using food as an emotional crutch, support can be invaluable in helping us deal with the feelings that come up.

Support comes in many different forms

We can ask other people or we can do it for ourselves; a mix of both is the best balance. Luana R., who came to a weekend workshop in London, has since set up an email group with other women from the same workshop. She has found it an invaluable way to stay connected. This is what she says about it:

❝ When one of the participants posts an email, others will reply back fairly quickly about how they have handled that particular situation if they have come across it and, possibly, some strategies they think might be useful. I know that, for me, it has been particularly useful when I have been struggling, though we have also written about our successes. To know that I can email the group with any concern and be met with unconditional support and useful strategies has been essential. 9

Whatever it looks like, support helps us to keep Beyond Chocolate alive rather than turning into another miracle solution that only lasts until the end of the book.

Ingrid Mouray, from London, did the 12-week multimedia course

6 Since following the Beyond Chocolate multimedia course in February 2005 I've carried on my journey of self-discovery by reading some of the books you've suggested, having four or five very useful sessions with a psychotherapist, and I joined a local support group.

It has been an amazing journey and still is. For the first time and for a whole six weeks from Christmas Eve I've been consistently eating when hungry, eating what I want, enjoying the food and stopping when full or satisfied. It is such a break-through. I've been feeling wonderful, light, slim (not just feeling it, the scales are saying the same thing), in tune with my body, I have forgotten the usual worries that I tend to have around food. It's been fantastic! 9

J.H., from Kingston, did a one-day workshop in London and the multimedia support

6 I have a deal now with a good friend: I bash out an email – I can type really fast so there is something quite satisfying about hitting the keys as I say it – and I put at the bottom "no reply

required". It seems quite funny really. I used it the other night after my ex had a go about how all my daughter's problems are my fault. I reacted like I used to, I didn't state my case, just sat and took on the rantings about my failings, and then I popped into my office bashed out how I felt with "no reply required". But my friend did reply – she always does – I got a text in the morning saying, "See just how far you have come and how he is still stuck". It works for me and within a very short period of time it had all dissipated, whereas before I could have literally dined out, and in, on that for weeks. ♪

ACTION!

A good place to start:

Signing up for the Beyond Chocolate Newsletter.

It's published every month and delivered by email. Full of practical tips and ideas, it's also absolutely free. It's an effortless source of support. We know that many women like to print it off and keep back issues around.

If you enjoy the interactive and immediate powers of the Internet, sign up to the Reader's Corner, on our website. This is a dedicated reader area where you can download more worksheets, audio activities and food for thought to support yourself along the way.

Put it on paper

Writing thoughts down in black and white helps you to formulate and understand them better. Keep a journal: you could write several pages every day, or dip in and out when you have something to say. You could buy yourself a beautiful notebook or use your PC – whatever works for you.

Reflection time

Set aside five minutes every day to tune in. Give yourself time to reflect on how you are doing, what you need and what you want.

Read all about it

Have a look at our Further reading (p. 241) for inspiring reads.

Close to home

Friends and family can offer a valuable listening ear, and it is a good idea to let the person who is willing to listen to you know that you don't expect her, or him, to fix the problem or to make it better and that you'll ask for advice if you want it. Sometimes simply hearing you out, listening to a good moan and providing a sounding board to help you unravel a challenging situation is the most positive kind of support.

Chocolate chums

Making changes on your own can be lonely, so ask a friend or colleague to do it with you. You can support and encourage each other and you'll have someone who knows what you're saying when you want to moan about how tough it can be and to celebrate with you when you feel on top of the moon.

Come on a Beyond Chocolate workshop

Have fun, meet interesting women, stimulate your grey cells and leave with all the practical strategies and tools you need – feeling nourished and empowered! That's what these women did:

❝ I have left this course with an array of strategies at my fingertips. I feel heard, supported, inspired and nourished. ❞
Eileen Williams, London

❝ A warm, welcoming environment, with great food, where you truly explore your relationship with food. ❞
Clair Ashford, Hertfordshire

❝ The weekend was an intensive investigation into my relationship with food, carried out in a supportive and nurturing environment. It has given me a way forward. ❞
Tracey Merrett, North Somerset

❝ I have really enjoyed myself. A lot of preparation and planning is evident, needed and works well. Very well thought-out course. ❞
Paula P., Hampshire

❝ A really well organised, well run and thought-out retreat, relaxing and nurturing. Pure bliss! I have really appreciated the attention to detail and the special little Beyond Chocolate touches. I have had a wonderfully relaxing, gently challenging time in such a warm and friendly atmosphere, with an emphasis on enjoyment and pleasure. I haven't felt so looked after since I was a little girl. ❞
Caroline McAdam, London

❛ The retreat was a wonderful, nurturing space in time, an opportunity in a shining setting to take stock of what really matters to me and to learn new skills. It has been fantastic. ❜

Sarah Layton, London

Have a look at the Beyond Chocolate workshops chapter (p. 223) for more information.

Psychotherapy

Today, therapy need not mean years of weekly sessions, lying on a couch. Short-term therapy with a specific focus is available and can be useful to support the work you have started by reading this book. There are many different kinds of therapy: humanistic, psychodynamic, gestalt, psychosynthesis, behavioural, analysis . . . and more. Finding the right type of therapist for you is important, so make sure that you take your time to choose. Have a face-to-face or phone conversation with the therapist before you make a decision. Let them know what you want from the sessions and find out how they work, what experience and training they have, and whether they are in supervision or work alone.

Personal development

There are many centres and organisations offering workshops and courses. Take care to find out as much about the organisation as possible before you commit yourself to anything. Look in the Chocolate Fairy's favourite resources (p. 215) to see the ones we can recommend from personal experience. If you are interested take a look at the following websites: www.spectrumtherapy.co.uk and www.transitions-europe.com.

REALITY CHECK

A study on support

In a study[1] carried out by nutrition researchers into supporting women with their food issues, women were divided into two groups: one group went on a standard weight loss diet, while the other group were told to let go of restrictive eating habits associated with dieting (similar to Beyond Chocolate). Instead they attended weekly support sessions and were invited to pay close attention to internal body cues indicating when they were truly hungry or satisfied, and to how they felt when they ate certain foods. The sessions were also designed to help them better understand their bodies and to become more accepting of them. They were encouraged to explore negative self-image, which might get in the way of them enjoying physical activity. After one year both groups showed similar improvements in metabolic fitness, psychology and eating behaviour. However half of the dieting group dropped out of the study, because, as we all know, it's impossible to stick to a diet for any length of time. Conversely, 92 per cent of the non-dieting group stayed in the study and were still going strong one year on. Support provided them with the motivation to keep going.

When we asked for help and let go of the restrictions and deprivations of dieting we can make long lasting changes rather than settling for quick-fix solutions which have us back to square one before we know it.

? DID YOU KNOW . . .

We humans are not designed to work alone. Successful people surround themselves with advisers and individuals who can offer them support. They make the decisions and they are in control, but they don't expect to do it all alone. Jesus had his twelve disciples, the PM has a cabinet and an endless posse of advisers, each an expert in their own field, entrepreneurs surround themselves with people who have the knowledge and experience they lack, chief executives have a board of directors. None of these people would dream of doing it alone or would see it as a weakness to ask for help.

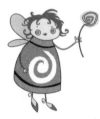

I taste the freedom when . . . I reach for the phone rather than the biscuit tin.

Food for thought

- How do you feel about asking for help?
- What are your beliefs about seeking professional help or support?
- What sources of support do you have at the moment?
- What kind of support would you like to have?
- How can you go about getting it?
- How will you support yourself?

Tune in

Eat when you are hungry

Eat whatever you want

Put it on a plate, sit down and focus

Stop when you are satisfied

Enjoy

Own your body

Move!

Support yourself

Be your own guru

CHAPTER 14

Who's the expert?

There is a mind-boggling array of weight-loss 'experts': doctors, celebrities, dieticians, TV chefs, newspaper columnists, slimming clubs and organisations, nutritionists, hypnotherapists, coaches, and so on. They all claim that they can tell you how to lose weight and that they know what's best. We have been told for so long that the experts know exactly what, when and how much we should eat, when in fact *we* are the only ones who have the answers to these questions. When we tune into our bodies, we find out what's best for us. We can become our own guru.

Before

I was always on the lookout for a new miracle that would change my life and make me thin. I really believed that the diet books or nutritionists, the doctors, the experts in magazines or the latest fitness fad held the answers I was looking for. I was convinced that if I did what they said I would become the slim, fit, attractive woman I so desperately wanted to be. I spent hours in the bookshops looking for the right diet and accumulated an impressive collection. I loved trying out the magazine diets, writing up weekly menus for myself and shopping to make sure I had everything I needed. I threw myself into these projects with utter conviction and I ended up doing the most ridiculous things on the say so of an expert. I really believed that they knew best.

I tried almost everything from slimming groups to holistic naturopaths. I took amphetamine-based pills to speed up my metabolism, prescribed quite legitimately by a dietician. I attempted to spend three weeks on a diet of meal replacements (except that I ended up eating all the chewy bars on the first day). I even tried surviving on a vile 'detox' concoction of warm water, lemon juice, maple syrup and cayenne pepper! I was willing to do the most absurd things in the hope of losing weight as long as it had the seal of approval of any kind of expert. It never even occurred to me for one moment that I might know what to do. I certainly didn't trust myself, even when the diets were not working.

Now

The first person I turn to for answers is me. I trust that I know what's best for me. I don't believe that because someone has a qualification or has written a book or made a television programme they know what I should and shouldn't be eating. I don't need to be told what to do, I find out for myself. I experiment, notice the results and learn from my experience. I have become my own guru.

What happened?

I read a book by Geneen Roth called *Breaking Free From Compulsive Eating* (now republished as *Breaking Free from Emotional Eating*), which confirmed my belief that diets don't work because they are one size fits all solutions. Diets are often touted as miracles. We are told that there is some intrinsic 'truth' to them and that the gurus who come up with them are somehow inspired. Letting go of the notion of needing 'experts' was such a challenge that for a while Geneen Roth became the expert I looked to along with Susie Orbach, Carol H. Munter, Naomi Wolf (see Further reading) and many more who all shared a similar philosophy. They all pointed me in the same direction: being curious about myself, learning more about what worked for me, making no assumptions, taking nothing for granted, being open to the unexpected, being willing to get messy and to make mistakes. I found out how much I needed to eat, what kinds of food satisfy me and what exercise to do to reach the weight that's just right for me, not by looking to an external qualified source but by listening to my body – which is infinitely more qualified to tell me about my needs.

What it boils down to

No one knows your body or what's right for it better than you do. You are the expert. That's not to say that we don't ever need professional help. Let's be clear about this: we are talking here about people who give weight-loss advice. Of course, if you have any kind of medical condition or special need, experts can be incredibly valuable and sometimes essential, but when it comes to weight loss *you* know best.

Think of the few women you know who are naturally slim, they don't do it by following expert advice, most of them have never been on a diet in their life. They instinctively know what they need and they trust those instincts. Becoming your own guru is about relearning to do just that. The reason why all our workshops are so successful is that Beyond Chocolate gives women back the power to make choices that really work for them, to learn how to listen to their bodies and to rebuild the trust in themselves that has been eroded by years of failed diets and eating plans dreamt up by others.

Being your own guru does not require qualifications, years of study or deep insights

It's about going back to basics. Eating is a biological need, just like going to the loo. Can you imagine being told when to go for a pee regardless of how much you've had to drink, when you drank it, and whether or not you feel like it.

No one has yet come up with a peeing plan because, luckily, we are still capable of knowing when we need to go. How do we do that? We recognise the signals and we know how to respond to them. Suggesting that others know when and how much you need to eat is just as ludicrous as the idea that someone else should tell us when and how often to pee.

Victoria, from London, did a weekend workshop in London

Before

❝ I always used to be about to start a diet, be on a diet or have just broken a diet. I thought if I could just "get slim" it would solve all my problems. I used to spend lots of money on slimming clubs, foods and books. I hated being weighed in public in front of everyone in the club. Before the weigh-in I would always go to the loo, wear my lightest clothes (never jeans), I even took off my jewellery. During the meeting I would plan my guilt-free blow out. I would go to the supermarket and buy chocolate and raisin pancakes. I'd eat the whole packet on the Tube on the way home. I couldn't stop and afterwards I would feel disgusted with myself. 〞

Now

〝 I spend my money on other things such as weekly fresh flowers and gorgeous moisturiser. I always have chocolate in the fridge and I can eat it anytime. I don't have to go through the humiliation of slimming clubs any more and I now have a free evening to pamper myself or catch up with friends. I have stopped the diet cycle and I feel FREE . . . I am now in control of the foods that I eat. I don't need to pay someone else to tell me which foods to put into my body. 〞

ACTION!

A good place to start:

Research . . . yourself!
Set aside some time to write about your relationship with food and your body on a regular basis. We are not suggesting you keep a food diary. This is something quite different. The focus here is on noticing, without criticism,

continued

the ways in which you use food in your life, how you feel about it and how your thinking goes. This is not about writing down every item that passes your lips every day. You don't have you fill reams and reams or have amazing insights – simply get into the habit of noticing yourself and being interested in who you are and what you do.

If you're sitting in front of a blank page, stuck for ideas, tune in. Jot down anything you notice and take it from there. For inspiration take a look at all the questions under Food for thought in the previous chapters.

Remember that you are a researcher and these are your field notes.

If it feels like homework

Buy yourself a notebook, one that's easy to carry around or looks good sitting on your desk. If you don't like hand-writing you could do it on your PC, and if you're a real web lover you could start a blog. If writing of any kind is not your thing, use a dictaphone or a camcorder, or just sit and reflect.

If you think you'll never have the time

You know best how long you'll need and will be willing to spend. It might be five minutes on the Tube, or it might be an hour at weekends, it might change depending on how you feel on any given day. If you're not sure, then experiment and find out what feels good. If you push yourself to do too much, you won't do it.

REALITY CHECK

A study on intuitive eaters

An American university professor carried out a study[1] with a group of college students who were naturally intuitive eaters and compared them to those who weren't. The students were then tested to see how healthy they were. Those who rated high on the intuitive eating scale were healthier than those who were at the bottom of the scale. He defines intuitive eating as: taking internal cues from the body, recognising what the body wants and then regulating how much you eat based on hunger and satiety rather than manipulating what we eat in terms of prescribed diets. He also suggests that long-term weight loss can be achieved while maintaining an unrestrained relationship with food. As he puts it 'As individuals get in touch with this "inner guide" or access their "inner wisdom" [that is, your own guru] they will be more in tune with the body's physical needs and will eat in a way that supports healthy weight maintenance and positive nutrition.'

 DID YOU KNOW . . .

More and more people are putting on weight despite the fact that there are more people following commercial diets and weight-loss programmes than ever before.

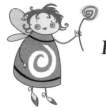

I taste the freedom when . . . I observe myself with gentle curiosity.

Food for thought

Time to think up your own . . .

CHAPTER 15

The two-letter word

Becoming a guru means redefining our relationship with food and our approach to weight loss. This might mean questioning and reformulating long-held beliefs. Saying yes to ourselves means that sometimes we say no to others. When we can say it with grace, confidence and assertiveness we can also say NO to food we don't want.

Before

I had rules and beliefs about everything from the way I should dress to the kinds of foods that I should or shouldn't eat. I had so many of them that I could have filled an encyclopaedia. I had very strongly held views about when it was OK to eat and when it wasn't, I was convinced that breakfast was the most important meal of the day, and if someone had gone to the trouble of cooking me a lovely meal it would have been the height of rudeness to refuse. Come to think of it, refusing any food I was offered was impolite. It was ungrateful and I might hurt the other person's feelings. I never questioned these beliefs, I just knew them, they were a part of me – they always had been. I lived by them, and when I lapsed I felt guilty. I never asked myself where I got them from and I did not stop to think if they were helpful or even true.

Some of them actually contradicted each other. I was too fat for fitted T-shirts that would have been vulgar and unsightly, but wearing baggy clothes was frumpy and unfeminine. I couldn't win. I believed that being thin was the answer to all my problems and that people who had willpower could stick to diets and lose weight forever. I was very critical of my shortcomings and I gave myself a really hard time. I had a nasty little voice in my head (aka the gremlin) that was very quick to point out when I transgressed and was always at hand to remind me how weakwilled and pathetic I was. It was exhausting.

Now

I still have enough beliefs to fill an encyclopaedia and I've thought about each one. The first one is that I don't beat myself up if I don't live by them. The second is that I'm open to changing them. I know that it's absolutely fine for me to say no to food that I don't want regardless of how much it cost, who prepared it, and what other people will think or say. I believe that comparing myself to anyone else is pointless and ultimately harmful. I know that when I use words such as 'I should', 'I ought to', 'I must', 'and I'll try', and 'I can't', I feel disempowered and ineffective. I am willing to risk upsetting someone if it means being true to myself. I update my beliefs regularly.

What happened?

I began to notice just how many rules and beliefs I churned out daily: from 'chocolate is evil' to 'you look tarty with makeup on'. Most of them were unhelpful and kept me stuck in the all-or-nothing mentality.

So I made a list. Here are just a few:

- It's not ladylike to have an appetite.

- I have to stay slim to keep my man.

- Women who want to be slim don't eat lunch.

- I should exercise for 45 minutes at least three times a week, or there's no point.

- You can't have your cake and eat it.

- My breasts are far too large.

- I shouldn't wear fitted T-shirts, I'm too fat.

- I mustn't say I don't like it, that's rude.

- I shouldn't say no.

- It's particularly ungrateful to say no to my aunt's casserole.

I could go on . . .

Sometimes I had no idea where they came from. Sometimes I could hear my mother's or my father's voice, echoing these comments and I began to wonder how I had made all these rules and beliefs for myself. I worked out where I had first heard them or seen them in action. I re-evaluated them, kept the ones that were helpful and ditched the ones that weren't and so I began to make my own beliefs. I based them on my experience of myself and my body and on my knowledge of what is helpful and unhelpful for me *now*. I also began to answer back when that voice in my head was on the attack. I put it in its place. Quickly and efficiently, no argument!

What it boils down to

Many of our beliefs and behaviours about food and our bodies come from our family, school, friends, media and society at large. They were passed on as verbal messages or through the way we saw adults around us behaving as we were growing up. As children, seeking love and approval, we tend to swallow them whole. When we're told that we have to clean the plate before we can leave the table, we do it, or get into trouble. If, as adults, we continue to eat everything that is on our plate, because that's 'what you do', we keep ourselves stuck with other people's rules, without giving ourselves the chance to find out what works for us.

Swallow and digest them, or spit them out

As adults we can decide what beliefs to believe in; we don't have to swallow them whole. It is interesting to see where specific messages come from because once we have identified them they are easier to deal with. Our parents most probably did their best; if they passed on unhelpful messages it's usually because they swallowed them whole, too. As adults we can choose what to believe, and, without pointing an accusatory finger, we can let go of old beliefs that do not belong to us and replace them with ones that work. How can we stop overeating if we always have to finish what's on our plate? Living by other people's rules means that we eat food we don't like, we eat more than we need, we squeeze ourselves into their expectations and ultimately stay stuck in the dieting rut.

When we start saying no to old beliefs we find that this sometimes means saying no to other people, like not eating at set meal times with family or friends, not going on a diet with our girlfriends, ordering the pasta when everyone else wants to share pizza. People can react defensively or aggressively to our 'no' and feel threatened or hurt. With a bit of practice, we can find ways of sticking to our beliefs without becoming rude or insensitive. When we stand firmly but gently by what works for us, we can accommodate other people's needs without sacrificing our own.

Pippa Kerslake, from London, did a weekend workshop in Dorset

Before

❛ My relationship with food used to fill me with such a negative guilty feeling. I used to say to myself: "No wonder you are overweight if you buy that" when I stood in a supermarket queue. "No wonder you are overweight if you eat that" when in a restaurant with friends.

I felt very self-conscious with friends and food. If there was a buffet I would have a battle in my head between what I thought I should choose and what I really wanted to choose. There wasn't much pleasure in food.

When I gave in and bought a large packet of crisps, or a pork pie, I would eat them in the car on the way home and put the empty packet in the outside bin so that it didn't count. I felt so guilty about what I'd done that I just carried on eating when I got home because I had ruined that day's "diet". I was so hard on myself. ❜

Now

❛ My relationship with food is now more relaxed. I enjoy food because I am tasting it, not gobbling it down with guilty feelings, and I have discovered that some of the food I used to categorise as "naughty" and so craved, like pork pies, I am not so keen on because it now tastes different.

Eating in a restaurant is much more about the social aspect, and I find choosing what I fancy easier. I realise that people are far more interested in themselves and what they choose to order and eat. It was me that used to judge myself so harshly, and now when that voice says, "You shouldn't eat that" I say, "Shut up, I can choose for myself." I hear that voice instead of thinking about what or when I am *meant* to eat.

Food has become a smaller part of my life; it takes up less of my head space. I feel lighter without the weight of guilt. ❜

ACTION!

A good place to start:

Update your beliefs.
Think of all the beliefs, rules and messages that you have about food and your body; write them down if you want to, and for each one ask yourself:

- Where or who did it come from?

- What decisions, conclusions or beliefs did I make about myself based on this message?

continued

- Is it helpful in any way?

- Do I want to keep it?

Now draw a line through all the ones you have decided get rid of.

   Example: *Women who want to be slim don't eat lunch.*

- Where did it come from?
  My mother.

- What decisions, conclusions or beliefs did I make about myself based on this message?
  That I should skip lunch if I want to lose weight.

- Is it helpful in any way?
  No, usually by mid afternoon I'm ravenous and I end up eating twice as much, and besides, by 3 pm my head is thumping and I can't concentrate on my work.

- Do I want to keep it?
  No thanks.

Saying no made simple

◉ When someone makes you an offer or asks something of you, it's always OK to ask for time to think about it. You don't have to agree to Sunday lunch straight away.

◉ When you say no make it assertive, look the person in the eyes. If you want to explain, keep it short and make it simple; for example, an assertive 'No thank you. I've had lunch already' works better than the over-apologetic 'Oh sorry, it looks really nice and I would but do you mind if I don't because I feel a bit full at the moment' or an aggressive 'Don't be ridiculous, there's no way I'm eating that, I had lunch half an hour ago.'

- Start the sentence with the word 'no', it's easier to stick with it if it's the first thing you say.

- Keep repeating your assertive, clear, polite 'No, thank you' until they get it.

- It takes practice, so start with some easy nos.

- Play a game. Choose a day when you will say yes and no truthfully, all day.

- Remind yourself that saying no to others means saying yes to yourself.

REALITY CHECK

Thanks but no thanks

Most people find it almost impossible to say 'No thanks' (eight letters). It's short, it's simple, it's to the point and we can use it to look after ourselves. So much easier than 'Oh thanks awfully but I couldn't possibly, well maybe just a little then' (58 letters!) or 'Yes, OK, I suppose that will be all right' (31 letters).

? DID YOU KNOW . . .

'It is a lot easier to say "no" to things you don't want to do if you have already said "yes" to things you do want to do.' Anonymous.

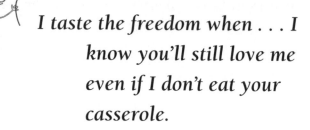

I taste the freedom when . . . I know you'll still love me even if I don't eat your casserole.

Food for thought

How often do you say yes when you mean no?

CHAPTER 16

Making it happen

If you want to stop yo-yo dieting, if you want a healthy relationship with food and your body, if you want to lose weight and keep it off, the only thing you *have* to do is take action. There are as many ways to take action as there are readers.

Start here

Let yourself off the 'weight-loss hook' for just a while. Beyond Chocolate is not a quick fix, you may not lose weight quickly, but when you do, it will be forever. Having weight loss as an objective is likely to sabotage your efforts. If for years you have been trying unsuccessfully to shed extra pounds, giving yourself some breathing space will provide you with an opportunity to road-test the only approach that can guarantee long-term success.

It's that easy. Once you have made a commitment to do something different, you can start to make changes, in whatever shape or form suits you best. The crucial thing to remember is that whatever small step you take, it's enough. As Goethe so pointedly says: 'Whatever you can do, or dream you can, *begin it!*' It is by taking a first, tiny step that we set in motion a chain reaction that soon has us running at full sprint. Somehow, the very fact that we have changed even just one thing opens a door and we start to see a whole host of new possibilities. There is no right way to get started. Make it as easy for yourself as possible. Start by experimenting with the principles you find the least challenging – there are lots of ideas in the Action! sections of each chapter. Integrate the others gradually as you feel more confident.

Which ones could you have a go at right now?

Beyond Chocolate Principles:

Tune in

Eat when you are hungry

Eat whatever you want

Put it on a plate, sit down and focus

Stop when you are satisfied

Enjoy

Own your body

Move!

Support yourself

Be your own guru

Start small and make it easy

Aiming to make huge changes all in one go often backfires. The idea is not to put this book down, vowing to follow the principles to the letter for ever and ever. If you are already thinking 'From now on, *every* time I eat I'm going to put the food on a plate, sit down and really focus on it' or 'I'm *never* going to eat when I'm not hungry again' STOP. You are set-ting yourself up for failure. The words 'every', 'never', 'always', and so on, imply that we cannot stray from a set course. This all-or-nothing approach, which is so dear to the diet mentality, keeps us stuck. When we get it wrong, we have failed and feel bad about ourselves and then we soon give up.

Take one day at a time. Decide that *today* you will eat one meal, sitting down and that you will really focus on it and that tomorrow you will pause for one minute when you find yourself about to eat and you know that you are not hungry. Every morning, when you wake up, decide on one action that you will take to do things differently; for example, Today I will . . .

- ⊚ eat one meal when I am hungry.

- ⊚ walk for ten minutes.

- ⊚ eat exactly what I want for dinner.

- ⊚ write in my journal for five minutes when I get the urge to eat and I know I'm not hungry.

- ⊚ stop when I'm satisfied when I go out to the restaurant tonight.

- ⊚ put my knife and fork down between each mouthful at one meal.

- ⊚ tune in before each meal.

Having one goal to focus on during the day makes it realistic and measurable. Each time you do it, you will feel good about yourself and be in the right frame of mind to keep going and doing things differently, rather than feeling constantly frustrated because you're not 'doing it all properly'. However busy you are, or whatever your lifestyle, you can do this. None of the above takes up a lot of time. You won't have to cook special meals or shop for a mind-boggling array of ingredients.

Appreciate yourself

Sometimes, even that one goal may prove to be more of a challenge than you had anticipated and you may not manage it. *That's OK!* The important thing is to notice as often as possible *how* you are approaching it. Are you resistant? Is it just too hard? Did you just plain forget? In fact, even if you just aim to notice when, what, why and how you eat for a while, without changing your current habits, you will be heading in the right direction and doing things differently already. Notice without criticism or judgement, and remember to put your gremlin in its place. The more you notice, the more information you will have and the easier it will be to make changes and to choose other objectives that you know you can do on other days. Every time you get to the end of a day and see that you have done something differently, appreciate yourself.

Go with the flow

Everyone has a different experience of Beyond Chocolate. You may start to lose weight steadily or you might put a little on before it goes for good. For a lucky few, it all falls into place rapidly. For most of us, transforming our approach to weight loss is a bumpy ride. You might do well for a while and then have periods where everything seems to be at a standstill. At other times, you may be managing one thing really well and find another aspect particularly challenging. You may occasionally feel rebellious, dejected or hesitant. This is completely normal – these are some of the phases that women go through on their way to a life Beyond Chocolate. These are the times when support can be especially helpful and valuable.

We have seen over and over again that our participants find the support crucial after the first few months. Finding a way to keep Beyond Chocolate alive, by talking about it with like-minded women, can make all the difference. Check out the Chocolate Fairy's favourite resources (p. 215), which are full of good ideas, and sign up to the Reader's Corner on our website to download extra materials. Use this book as a reference. If you have someone to do Beyond Chocolate with, then so much the better.

In a nutshell

- Beyond Chocolate is not a set of rules or guidelines. You cannot do it right or wrong; everything you do, every step you take, has something valuable to teach you.

- Be curious about yourself – ask lots of questions and be willing to reconsider old beliefs and rules that no longer work for you.

- Be interested in why you do things and how you do them – observe yourself with curiosity as if you were conducting an experiment on a fascinating subject (you!). Notice if you judge or criticise yourself for the way that you eat or the way your body looks and remind yourself that in the context of this experiment there is no right or wrong, just interesting.

- Make changes slowly, one bite at a time – the way you work towards your goal is as important as getting there.

- Be open to what you will discover, your destination may be even better than you had imagined!

- No one method can work for everyone. Each one of us needs a personally designed, perfectly suited system and the *best* person to discover what yours looks like is you.

- Dieting and deprivation takes effort, willpower and determination – Beyond Chocolate takes willingness, commitment and curiosity.

- Come back to this chapter whenever you need to remind yourself how to do it!

Cathie Wilson, from Herefordshire, did a weekend workshop in Gloucestershire and the multimedia course

How a Brussels sprout sums up the Beyond Chocolate way:

❝ I have been eating everything that I love for over a year: mascarpone cheese, bacon rind, toast and butter, peanut butter . . . and Brussels sprouts. I discovered that I positively longed for Brussels sprouts – especially with Parmesan cheese . . . or melted butter . . . or black pepper. I cannot believe that for so long I didn't eat them, even though I love them.

Beyond Chocolate has helped me to recognise and acknowledge so many issues that I now know *why* I didn't eat them: no one in my family likes them. So I didn't buy them. Beyond Chocolate teaches you to listen to yourself (yes, I like Brussels sprouts). It teaches you to value yourself (yes, I can spend some of the family budget on food that only I like). It teaches you to eat what you want, even if it is socially awkward

("Are you really going to eat just sprouts for tea?" – actually no one has noticed my sprout habit!). It teaches you to leave your past behind (my mother's Brussels sum up all that is awful in old-fashioned cooking). It teaches you to value the quality of your food (I have tried so many different retailers, as I experiment with different types of sprouts). It gives you back joy in food! (Yeehay! Sprouts are in season!)

The other day on the radio I heard a dietician say the words "eating what you want and when you are hungry is a recipe for getting fat". It shocked me back into the groove. My brain added "– in the short term" because I know that my weight has been stable for over a year. I do not weigh an ounce more.

My friend, who I have encouraged but not succeeded in converting to the Beyond Chocolate way, has spent a year of managing her weight in different ways, with the result that she is back where she began. I have listened while she complained about points, counted carbs, plodded through diet drinks, and ate a salad when the weather was cold and when it really called for a baked potato. I've had so much pleasure, while she has been so sad. That's the difference the Beyond Chocolate way makes. 〞

Everyone can do Beyond Chocolate

We all have what it takes to go back to basics and listen to our bodies. And it's not hard. You don't need willpower, you don't need to deprive yourself, you don't have to follow any rules and you don't need to listen to others. You are your own guru.

Ultimately, a life Beyond Chocolate is a life of freedom. Imagine a life where you get up in the morning without automatically thinking about your weight and what you are going to eat or *not* going to eat that day. A life when you can't remember the last time you even considered dieting. A life where you sit down to meals knowing that you are about to eat exactly what you fancy, that no food is forbidden or bad. Imagine a life where food and eating are associated with pleasure and fun. A life where you know just how much it takes for you to be perfectly satisfied and contented. A life where you get pleasure from wearing clothes that you feel really good in. Where you feel the benefits of moving your body *and* enjoy it. A life where you know where to turn when the going gets tough, trusting that you will receive support. A life where your self-esteem does not depend on your weight but on the real you. A you who has more energy, time and money to dedicate to things that truly nourish you. A you who is confident and shines out to the world.

You can start to taste that freedom now. Welcome to your life Beyond Chocolate.

CHAPTER 17

FAQs: Yes, but . . . what if?

On our workshops and in response to our newsletter we are asked lots of questions. Here are some of the ones that pop up most frequently.

Q: There are so many programmes and diets out there, why is Beyond Chocolate any different?

A: There is *nothing* like Beyond Chocolate available in the UK. Beyond Chocolate wasn't created to make money, it was born from the passion of two real women's experiences. We know what you're talking about because we've been there. We give you *real* solutions to *real* problems. This book is the fruit of our experiences, not just a theory. You won't have to change to fit our programme, you can take the principles and fit them into your life in a way that works for you.

Most programmes provide you with a set of one-size-fits-all answers. No other book tells you to trust yourself. We know that you have all the answers you need, we are simply guiding you towards them. We also keep our workshops small rather than cramming hundreds of participants into a day, so that each woman has an opportunity to discover the strategies that will work for her.

Q: I've read so many weight-loss books, I'm usually inspired and quite fired up for a few weeks and then the effects wear off and I'm back where I started. Isn't this going to be the same?

A: We are not simply interested in selling you an inspiring book. We know that to make lasting changes you will need encouragement and there is an organisation behind this book to provide support and motivation. You can log on free of charge to the Reader's Corner on our website for lots more practical tools and strategies, sign up for our free monthly newsletter or come on a workshop.

Q: You say that Beyond Chocolate is not about willpower but surely we will need willpower to stop us from just eating when we should be stopping and thinking about why we want to eat first?

A: No, with Beyond Chocolate you won't need willpower at all. Willpower is self-defeating when it comes to stopping overeating. If you rely on willpower, which in this case means resisting the urge to overeat, eventually you will get to the flip side of resisting, which is giving in and overeating in a big way! Remember, we are not suggesting that you 'should' be stopping and thinking why you want to eat. Words like 'should', 'ought to' and 'must' are unhelpful and you won't find them in this book. They imply that there is a right way to do things, and if there's a right way then there's also a wrong way, but when you think you are doing it wrong you're likely to not do it at all, which takes us straight back to that unhelpful all-or-nothing diet mentality.

Instead of thinking that you 'should' stop overeating, start by doing exactly the opposite. Allow yourself to do it, and when you do, aim to notice as much as you can about how you feel, what you do and what led you to it. When you acknowledge that overeating is the way you know, at the moment, to comfort yourself or distract yourself or give yourself a treat (or whatever it is for you) you will be in control and you'll learn something of value. When you are in control you can decide to stop when you are ready. Not because you are using every ounce of willpower you have to hold yourself back, but because you can find a way of meeting your needs that does not involve food. This is a gradual process – take another look at Chapters 5 and 16 to remind you just how to go about it.

Q: You always refer to women in this book and never to men; can Beyond Chocolate work for men too?

A: Yes I'm sure it can. Both men and women overeat. In our society there is added pressure on women (though sadly I think men are catching up quickly) to be thin and beautiful. As women we define ourselves by how we look, we equate being successful with being thin and being attractive. We feel good about ourselves if we look good. Most men still define themselves by their jobs, their financial status or their sportsmanship. Anyone who overeats uses food to fill a gap – men and women alike. We haven't had men on the workshops so we can't say for sure but we can see no reason why they should not be able to benefit from the Beyond Chocolate principles.

Q: I am diabetic (or have a food intolerance/allergy), does that mean that Beyond Chocolate is not for me?

A: You *can* integrate all the Beyond Chocolate principles into your life if you are diabetic or have food intolerances or allergies. Eating what you want does not mean ignoring your health and safety. If you are diabetic and eating foods high in sugar sends you into insulin shock then you can look after yourself and choose to eat whatever foods you want that you can eat *safely*. If in doubt, consult your doctor before making any changes.

You may well have strong feelings about not being able to eat all the foods you want and you might even find yourself craving the very foods you can't have. If you acknowledge those feelings rather than telling yourself you shouldn't feel like that because it's pointless, you are likely to find it easier not to eat the foods that aren't safe for you.

Eating what we want is about listening to our bodies, and if your body is sending you a clear signal that certain foods are harmful then you can learn to listen and respond appropriately, knowing that you are looking after yourself.

Q: The problem is I get so depressed about the way I look I just can't see beyond that and it makes me eat more for comfort, I suppose. I know that you can't guarantee that this approach will work but can you just give me an idea of the likelihood of it succeeding so that I won't feel as if I have failed if I don't tune in or follow the principles a few times?

A: When participants come to our workshops almost all of them want to know how long the process will take, how soon they'll lose weight. By the end of a workshop they know that there is so much more to it than the size of their body. Weeks or months later they measure success not by the amount of weight they've lost or how well they are sticking to the principles – they talk about feeling free, about understanding themselves better, about having bigger, brighter lives. We cannot guarantee how much weight you will lose or how long it will take – what we *can* tell you is that if you are willing to experiment with the principles we've outlined in this book, if you are prepared to listen to yourself and live in the present – today, as you are right now – then you cannot fail.

Q: You say that we can eat what we like, but it might take us months before we settle down to healthy eating. Surely we should be aiming for healthy eating sooner rather than later?

A: Yes, it could well take months. We all have a different pace. If you know that aiming for healthy eating helps you have a healthy balanced diet all the time, that's all well and good. If, on the other hand, aiming for 'healthy eating' keeps you stuck in an endless all-or-nothing cycle then it's clearly not healthy in the long run. Beyond Chocolate is about being healthy all round and not just for a few weeks: by eating foods that leave you feeling nourished and satisfied when you're hungry, by using your body to move and feel fit, by having a healthy attitude towards your body and by being willing to find out and experience what is really going on instead of overeating. Aiming for a healthy attitude to food will get you to a healthy diet – it may take a little longer but it will last a lifetime.

Q: I would find it very difficult to buy lots and lots of one of my forbidden foods and then see them go to waste if I go off them. Can't I buy a little at a time?

A: The simple answer to that is NO. If you buy just a little then it will be all too tempting to finish it off. If you haven't allowed yourself this food 'legally' for a while, having just a little will feel like a treat and it will be hard to know how much is enough. You might feel tempted to eat it all in one go, so that it's gone and you don't have to face it again. Or you might finish it all and still not feel satisfied . . . which might leave you feeling like a bottomless pit. Participants on our workshops often find they need to buy much more than they initially thought (and sometimes more than they felt comfortable with to begin with) to be in a position to decide when to stop. So, if you're worried about wasting food think about what you'll do with any leftovers – look back over Chapter 8 for some ideas.

Q: I would love to buy some really nice clothes that would fit me just as I am so that I would feel good about myself, but deep down I keep thinking what a waste it will be to spend all the money on clothes that, hopefully, won't fit me in a few months. I have to work very hard for the money I earn. I just don't feel right about it. What can you suggest I do, or should I just try to change my mindset about that?

A: Beyond Chocolate is not about trying to change your mindset. There is nothing that you 'should' do; only choices that you can make if you want to. If you feel uncomfortable buying some really nice new clothes then what would feel OK? Would you be willing to go through your wardrobe and pack up all the clothes that don't fit – either because they're too tight or too big – and put them away, out of sight? When you've done that, take a look at what is left. If it's enough to be getting on with, until you feel ready to buy some new clothes, that's fine. If you need a few more items then could you get just a few things that wouldn't cost an arm and a leg or that you could still wear even when you do lose weight? When we continue to live for tomorrow, for what we will be one day, we miss out on living now. We can spend our whole lives putting everything on hold, waiting, because tomorrow we will be ready, when we are thin, when everything is just right. You can start to live today, whatever your budget or your size.

Q: You say to take time to tune in before eating, but part of me just wants to eat then and there, so I would find it really hard to stop and tune in. Perhaps it just takes practice.

A: Yes, it all just takes practice and willingness. Tuning in takes just a minute or less, and the more you do it the easier and quicker it gets. To start with, it can be just as helpful to notice when you do find yourself rebelling and unwilling to stop for even that minute. Keep on noticing and keep on aiming to tune in – eventually you will. Awareness is 50 per cent change!

Q: I have never really taken much exercise and I would feel so awful and silly exercising while I'm still overweight, although I know that moving around will be good for me. I couldn't possibly join an exercise class and feel that a few minutes of jumping around at home won't make any difference.

A: You are absolutely right that moving will be good for you. Even ten minutes jumping around at home is a step closer to being fit than nothing at all. It *all* makes a difference. If you don't feel comfortable joining an exercise class and if dancing around your living room just isn't your thing, that's fine – what would you feel comfortable doing? You will only do it if it is tolerable at the very least, so think about what you are willing to do. Would you go for a ten-minute walk? It's the easiest way to start. All you need is a pair of comfortable walking shoes. If you enjoy it you can gradually walk for longer and more often. Have another look at Chapter 12 for some more ideas.

Notes

Chapter 1

1 Polivy, J., 'Psychological consequences of food restriction', *Journal of the American Dietetic Association*, 96, 1996, pp. 589–92.

Chapter 3

1 Food and Agriculture Organization (FAO) of the United Nations.

Chapter 4

1 Corinne Marmonier, Didier Chapelot, Marc Fantino and Jeanine Louis-Sylvestre, 'Snacks consumed in a nonhungry state have poor satiating efficiency: influence of snack composition on substrate utilization and hunger', *American Journal of Clinical Nutrition*, 2002, Vol. 76, pp. 518–28.

Chapter 5

1 Cesar G. Fraga, 'Cocoa, Diabetes and Hypertension: should we eat more chocolate?', Department of Nutrition, University of California, Davis, and Physical Chemistry-PRALIB (CONICET), University of Buenos Aires, Argentina, *American Journal of Clinical Nutrition*, Vol. 81 (3), 2005, pp. 541–2.

2 Marcia Levin Pelchat, Andrea Johnson, Robin Chan, Jeffrey Valdez and J. Daniel Ragland, 'Images of desire: food-craving activation during fMRI', *NeuroImage*, Vol. 23, 2004, pp. 1486–93.

3 Christine L. Pelkman, et al., 'Reproductive hormones and eating behavior in young women', *American Journal of Clinical Nutrition*, Vol. 73, 2001, pp. 19–26.

Chapter 6

1 Jean L. Kristeller and C. Brendan Hallett, 'An exploratory study of a meditation-based intervention for binge eating disorder', Department of

Psychology, Indiana State University, *Journal of Health Psychology*, Vol. 4 (3), 1999, pp. 357–63.

2 Ibid.

Chapter 7
1 Samara Joy Nielsen and Barry M. Popkin, 'Patterns and trends in food portion sizes, 1977–1998', *The Journal of the American Medical Association*, 289, 2003, pp. 450–3.

2 Nicole Diliberti, Peter L. Bordi, Martha T. Conklin, Liane S. Roe and Barbara J. Rolls, 'Increased portion size leads to increased energy intake in a restaurant meal', Department of Nutritional Sciences and School of Hotel, Restaurant, and Recreation Management, The Pennsylvania State University.

3 B. Burton-Freeman, P. Davis and B. Schneeman, 'Cholecystokinin is asso ciated with subjective measures of satiety in women', *Plasma American Journal of Clinical Nutrition*, Vol. 76 (3), 2002, pp. 659–67.

Chapter 10
1 We have spent months researching this subject in the search for a definitive answer. We haven't found one. The research and evidence is so conflicting, we have found as many studies that say it's unhealthy to be overweight as those that say that size, in all but extreme cases, has no impact on our health.

2 Sherry Turner, Heather Hamilton, Meija Jacobs, Laurie M. Angood & Deanne Hovde Dwyer, 'The influence of fashion magazines on the body image satisfaction of college women: An exploratory analysis', *Adolescence*, 32 (127), 1997, pp. 603–13.

Chapter 12
1 Dallas Cooper Institute, Aerobics Center Longitudinal Study.

2 S. N. Blair, H. W. Kohl III, C. E. Barlow, R. S. Paffenbarger Jr, L. W. Gibbons, and C. A. Macera, 'Changes in physical fitness and all-cause mortality', *Journal of the American Medical Association*, Vol. 273, 1995, pp. 1093–8.

3 See also Paul Campos, *The Obesity Myth: Why America's Obsession with Weight is Hazardous to Your Health*, Gotham Books, 2004, pp. 35–6.

Chapter 13

1 L. Bacon, N. L. Keim, M. D. Van Loan, M. Derricote, B. Gale, A. Kazaks and J. Stern, 'Evaluating a "non-diet" wellness intervention for improvement of metabolic fitness, psychological well-being and eating and activity behaviors', *International Journal of Obesity*, Vol. 26 (6), 2002, pp. 854–65.

Chapter 14

1 Steven R. Hawks, Hala Madanat, Jaylyn Hawks and Ashley Harris, 'The relationship between intuitive eating and health indicators among college women', *Journal of Health Education*, November 2005.

Log on for more

We love the Internet. Thanks to email, blogs, newsletters, forums and networks we can all have our say and become 'gurus'. Thanks to the Internet our participants can stay in touch with us long after they have attended a workshop; it's so much easier to dash off a quick email or to post a few words on the forum than finding time to write a letter and stick it in the post. We're delighted that we have subscribers and multimedia course participants from as far away as Australia to just across the Channel, which means we can start to expand our horizons and support more and more women in other places – watch out for *Au Delà du Chocolat*!

We are really excited about our new Reader's Corner. If you are an Internet user and like to get interactive, you can access this specially dedicated reader area on our website. Go to www.beyondchocolate.co.uk and click on Reader's Corner on the homepage. When you register you will be asked for a password, type in: MORECHOCOLATE

Here's what you'll find in the Reader's Corner:

All the worksheets and written exercises that are included in this book If you're like us and have always had an aversion to writing in books, you can download the worksheets and exercises, and print them off instead. Even if you have filled in the worksheets in the book, this is a good opportunity to do some of them again at a later date. It's amazing to see how we evolve at different stages in our relationship with food and our bodies. Print them off or save them on your computer and keep them to hand so that you can use them when in need of inspiration, motivation and further reflection.

New worksheets and written exercises We are constantly updating our materials as we learn more, experiment with new ideas and receive inspiring feedback from Beyond Chocolate 'gurus'. Log on to keep up with new ideas.

Audio material Download our audio files on to your computer and even on to your iPod so that you can access Beyond Chocolate whenever you need it and wherever you are. Guided audio activities to get you thinking, inspiring dialogues and music to get you moving! No chanting, tapping or hypnosis techniques; just straightforward questions to help you gather information and get your imagination going.

Links to great resources You will find websites that offer useful and practical products, and services that we have found helpful, as well as Beyond Chocolate (and non-chocolate) events where you can meet like-minded women and have fun.

Reader's Corner . . . chapter by chapter

Once you have registered, you can click straight on to each *Beyond Chocolate* chapter title in the Reader's Corner to:

LOG ON FOR MORE • 211

A life beyond chocolate

Register on the Reader's Corner and take an easy step towards your life Beyond Chocolate.

The all-or-nothing trap

Beyond Chocolate celebrates 'no diet day' on 6 May. Log on to our website to find out what we have in store.

Back to basics

Download and print off the 'Beyond Chocolate Principles in a Nutshell' sheet. Use it as a bookmark or stick it into your diary as a gentle reminder of your commitment and intentions.

Save that slice of cake for later, when you're hungry

What are you really hungry for? Download this guided audio activity and find out.

The answer to a problem is not always a cup of tea and a biscuit . . . or ten

Next time you find yourself reaching for a chocolate bar and you know you're not hungry, reach for your mouse instead and download an audio activity that will certainly give you food for thought.

Chocolate sandwiches for breakfast

Do you think chocolate is evil, ice cream is irresistible and chips are dangerous? Do this exercise to find out more about your forbidden foods and their personalities. The more you do it, the more fun it gets.

Eating crisps by candlelight

For a true slow-food experience, download this audio activity armed with some of your favourite chocolate. Our guided tasting session will take you through some simple steps to discover the taste of your favourite food.

Just how much is enough?

Full or satisfied, that's the question. It's different every time, and for each one of us. Do this worksheet as often as you like, and find out which is which.

You are not a dustbin

Listen to a discussion about waste that will get you thinking.

Eating chocolate, without the guilty aftertaste

We have made it our mission over the years to seek out the yummiest, most mouth-watering food out there. Log on to our website for links to the best gourmet goodies we have found.

Mirror, mirror on the wall

Is there any way in which it's helpful to be the size you are? Does focusing all your energy on weight loss mean that you can avoid dealing with other problems? Find out more by logging on and doing this gently challenging audio activity.

Every item in my wardrobe fits just right

Shopping for clothes doesn't have to be a thankless task. Find out how to make it a fun and fruitful day.

Work it out

Log on to our website and find out how you can start getting fit even if you can spare only eight minutes. Download Gabrielle Roth's 5Rhythms Warm Up and start moving rather than exercising.

Asking for help, not a second helping

What is support and how do we go about getting it? Download this article and find out more about it.

Who's the expert?

If you're stuck for inspiration, download more Food for thought.

The two-letter word

Download some helpful worksheets on saying no and up-dating your beliefs.

Making it happen

Receive a daily Chocolate Fairy in your inbox with useful Action! suggestions and Food for thought.

Yes, but . . . what if?

Log on to our website to see more answers to questions that have been asked by Beyond Chocolate participants. Send us your questions and we'll print them in our newsletter.

The Chocolate Fairy's favourite resources

Most of the resources are London based but they all offer online access. If you have a fantastic resource elsewhere in the UK (or even abroad), we'd love to hear from you.

Organisations we can recommend

Spectrum This Humanistic training centre and practice offers lots of ways to approach self-development, from individual therapy to numerous workshops on every topic you can think of (anger, sexuality, self-esteem, couples, parenting, and so on). The structure of the organisation ensures a highly professional and ethical service.
Website: www.spectrumtherapy.co.uk
Address: 7 Endymion Road, London, N4 1EE
Tel: 020 8341 2277

BACP (The British Association for Counselling and Psychotherapy) A good starting place to find a therapist, BACP is UK wide, so it is useful if you don't live in London. The organisation sets, promotes and maintains standards for the counselling profession. It publishes a Counselling and

Psychotherapy Resources Directory (CPRD), a comprehensive list of counsellors, psychotherapists, supervisors, trainers, organisations and services available. BACP has published guidance to members of the public on choosing the most appropriate counsellor or psychotherapist according to their needs.
Website: www.bacp.co.uk

Woman Within Every woman who participates in a Woman Within Training Weekend gets just what she went there for, be it connection with other women, empowerment, self-awareness and esteem, fun and laughter . . . The workshops are inspiring and life changing, and there's even a brother organisation called the Mankind Project for your partners, husbands, sons, brothers, and so on.
Websites: www.womanwithin.org
www.transitionseurope.com

Triyoga We love the atmosphere in these London-based centres offering classes on yoga, meditation and Pilates as well as a whole range of holistic treatments from truly qualified professionals. There's something for everyone: from pregnancy meditation for couples to weekend workshops on yoga to awaken the body, and foundation Pilates courses. It makes the whole 'yoga' scene accessible, thanks to friendly staff, inspiring classes and affordable prices – a great place to start taking care of your body and soul. Triyoga has centres in Primrose Hill, Soho and Covent Garden in London.
Website: www.triyoga.co.uk

British Wheel of Yoga We'd love Triyoga to open up all over the UK, but sadly they are only in London at the moment. There are lots of great yoga teachers all over the country and The British Wheel of Yoga is a good place to look for a class in your area, wherever you live. Log on to their website or give them a call. They can recommend a trained yoga teacher who runs classes near you. You could try your local sports centre, too, they often have yoga classes that are convenient and affordable.

Website: www.bwy.org.uk

Tel: 01529 306851

Other women doing stuff we love

Here are the other women who are doing stuff we love – to nourish your mind, body and soul.

Surinder Phull is Head Nutritionist at Eat Well Nutrition Consultancy. We love her holistic, no-diet approach to nutrition and eating, and she regularly contributes to our newsletter with cutting-edge nutritional news and unconventional ideas. If you would like to discover more about how your body and your health are impacted by the foods you eat – without the words 'calories' and 'weight loss' ever being mentioned – she is the person to turn to. Surinder is available for private consultations throughout London and across the UK.

Website: www.eatwell.co.uk

Veronica Lim offers a very Beyond Chocolate-like approach to managing your money. Her Millionaire Thinking for Women workshop was insightful and full of useful, practical tools. If you want to free yourself from constantly worrying about your finances, contact Veronica for more information on her tailor-made workshops and coaching.

Email: veronica@veronicalim.com

Sue Rickards runs 5Rhythms dance classes, workshops and retreats for anyone who wants to dance – even if you imagine you're too young, old, unfit, small, big, nervous, inexperienced, disabled or shy. 5Rhythms is simple, joyous and a great way of moving your body – and the beauty of it is that, like Beyond Chocolate, you can't get it wrong! Or right, for that matter – it's a chance to explore for yourself, whatever limitations or experience you have. Bring out the dance guru in you. Sue's website also offers links to other 5Rhythms teachers and classes across the UK and abroad.

Website: www.acalltodance.com

Kira Balaskas is the person we turn to for a truly different massage experience. Kira has been practising and teaching Thai Yoga Massage in London since 1989 and is recognised by the International Society of Thai Yoga Massage. In this wonderful head-to-toe massage, the practitioner uses her hands, feet and elbows to apply pressure to different parts of your body in combination with gentle stretching and applied yoga postures. This blissful two-hour massage leaves you feeling deeply relaxed or incredibly energised, depending on your needs and also has healing qualities for all kinds of aches and pains. A cross between yoga and massage, it's a great way of moving your body! Find a qualified practitioner near you on Kira's website.

Website: www.thaiyogamassage.co.uk

OK, so he's not a woman but . . .

Gareth Williams is our resident yoga teacher and Thai Massage Therapist on our Retreats. We love his approach to yoga, which he says many women avoid because they think they have to be flexible, fit, young or slim to be able to do it. As Gareth says 'There is so much more to yoga than getting into bizarre twisted positions . . . whoever you are, you can benefit from practising a yoga that is appropriate for you!' He runs yoga classes in Cheltenham, Tewkesbury and London, and roams the UK to deliver fantastic Thai Yoga Massage (not surprising, he trained with Kira!).

Email: gareth@livingyoga.org.uk

Where to buy great chocolate

When we started to really taste the food we were eating and took time to savour every bite, Mars Bars and Green & Black's just didn't satisfy our taste buds any longer. It only took one bite of Rococo's magic chocolate to open the door to a whole new world. Since then, one of our favourite pastimes is seeking out new chocolate sensations. There are so many, and we are constantly discovering more. Here are just a few that we can personally recommend.

Rococo Chocolates We love Chantal Coady's approach to making chocolate. Her handmade, organic, Fairtrade gems are fantastic. Whether you are biting into one of her orgasmic saffron and cardamom truffles or breaking off a piece of any one of her fabulous artisan bars (our current favourites are dark chocolate with geranium and orange, and white chocolate with cardamom) the experience is luxurious, sensual and an explosion for your taste buds. Order online or wander about her beautifully decorated London shops at 45 Marylebone High St, London W1U 5HG and 321 Kings Road, London SW3 5EP.

Website: www.rococochocolates.com

Seventypercent.com Welcome to the world of real chocolate! A one-stop shop for all your chocolate needs. News, reviews and articles on the world's finest chocolates, all the big names are there. Amongst our favourites: Amedei, Bonnat, Domori, Cluizel. Buy them bar by bar or sign up to the Chocolate Connoisseur Club and get a selection delivered to your door every month.

Website: www.seventypercent.com

Pierre Marcolini Seriously the *best* filled chocolates we have ever tasted! These melt-in-the-mouth little luxuries combine the most astonishing flavours for a real knock-out effect – expensive and lavish but well worth it. Visit the shop at 6 Lancer Square, London W8 4EH or order online.

Website: www.pierremarcolini.co.uk

The Chocolate Society Out and about and fancy something chocolatey? The Chocolate Society shops stock all types of chocolate, from bars to truffles, plus everything in between, from chocolate liqueur to brownies, ice cream and milkshakes – all made with quality chocolate. And they even have café areas with tables where you can sit down, put it on a plate and really enjoy the experience. Visit their shops at 36 Elizabeth Street, London SW1W 9NZ and 32–34 Shepherd Market, London W1J 7QN, or order online.

Website: www.chocolate.co.uk

Day Chocolate Company The Divine and Dubble ranges of Fairtrade chocolate not only taste good but are also helping women in Ghana to support their families and educate their children. It's very affordable and you can buy it at your local Tesco or Sainsbury's.

The Chocolate Fairy's little luxuries

When we stopped dieting and stepped off the weight-loss treadmill, we discovered that we had more time, more energy and more money to spend on things that truly nourished us.

These are just some of our favourites that we have picked up over the years.

Natural Magic Candles We burn one at the Beyond Chocolate office and it is absolutely amazing. Made with natural vegetable wax and 100 per cent pure essential oils, they burn without releasing harmful pollutants and smell just heavenly. Instructions: Light the candle; kick off your shoes and sit or lie down somewhere comfortable; close your eyes; breathe in the wonderful fragrances and melt away for just ten minutes. A delicate scent will linger in the air throughout the day. At £35 a candle it is expensive, but the candle burns for 50 hours, that's 300 days' worth of ten-minute breaks in a year.

Website: www.naturalmagicuk.com

The Body Shop Home Fragrance Oil A few drops of 'line-dried cotton' oil in a burner fills our kitchen with the smell of fresh laundry, even when we've used the tumble dryer – the Body Shop makes lots of these home fragrance oils, and they don't cost an arm and a leg.

L'Occitane's Honey Incense Sticks Burn one of these in your kitchen and it smells like you've been baking honey cake. £12 for 40 sticks – that's a lot of honey cakes!

Website: www.loccitane.com

The Sanctuary Footcare Pamper Kit At £5 and from any Boots store, this little box is heaven for our feet, especially after we've run a workshop. The Foaming Pumice Foot Scrub and Soothing Foot Soufflé are perfect for tired tootsies and you even get a buffer and nail file to make them shine beautifully.

Palais des Thés Look here for 230 teas from more than 25 countries around the globe, as well as good ethics, beautiful packaging, delicate little muslin tea bags and exquisite tea accessories. We love the Palais des Thés, which unfortunately still hasn't opened shops in the UK. If you are in Paris you can see for yourself or you can browse through and order from the vast online catalogue. Our favourite? Ikebana: a flowery blend of green and black tea with mint, rose, jasmine and orchid. Brew a pot and take five minutes to sit and enjoy the enticing aroma.

Website: www.le-palais-des-thes.fr

Angel Cards We like starting our day by picking one of these tiny, fun cards that come in a deck of 72. Each card contains a word and an illustration that provide an inspiring thought for the day or it can be used for meditation.

Website: www.innerlinks.com

Beyond Chocolate workshops

One-day workshop An introduction to Beyond Chocolate, which brings this book to life and gives you the opportunity to experience the principles first-hand.

Multimedia course Ideal if you can't get away for a workshop. Weekly emails, audio CD, telephone consultation, access to the forum for ongoing support and lots of useful little gifts (plus optional individual or group support sessions in London).

Weekend workshops Join us in a beautiful country setting for a 'get away from it all' nurturing experience with fabulous food, or in London for a non-residential weekend. Both are full immersion, experiential workshops with plenty of time for personalised guidance.

Retreats in Italy A week-long intensive course in a fabulous setting amid the olive groves of Puglia – Italy's new Tuscany. Combine a creative, empowering workshop with a nurturing holiday: beauty treatments, yoga, swimming, cultural activities, walks and divine meals. No one shares a room in this boutique hotel with a private pool; everyone has their own gorgeous en-suite bedroom.

Support sessions These are open to any Beyond Chocolate workshop participant, and they provide the opportunity to stay motivated and supported. Evenings in London, multi-media support, phone consultations or individual sessions.

More information on Beyond Chocolate workshops is available at www.beyondchocolate.co.uk

Or contact:
    Beyond Chocolate
    PO Box 56905
    London
    N10 2YN
    Tel: 020 8883 0472

Guru work

Worksheet 1:
YOUR EXPERT OPINION

You are your own guru. Only you know what is right for you, what will work and how you can fit Beyond Chocolate into your life so that it is doable and enjoyable. **We cannot stress this enough.**

So many different women have come on our workshops: some are nursing mothers, some have diabetes, some are physically impaired or suffer from illnesses, others are going through a particularly hectic moment in their lives. They all have different needs.

Take a look at the ten principles below and for each one make a note of:

◉ *Your immediate reaction*

◉ *What obstacles you see coming up*

◉ *Is there one principle that stands out that you think might be particularly challenging?*

◉ *Are there any that you already practise?*

◉ *Is there is one or more that you think will prove difficult, challenging or impractical because of your specific needs and lifestyle?*

Beyond Chocolate Principles

Tune in

Eat when you're hungry

Eat whatever you want

Put it on a plate, sit down and focus

Stop when you're satisfied

Enjoy

Own your body

Move!

Support yourself

Be your own guru

Which principles can you do now?

You are your own guru, *you* know what will and what won't work. Focus on the principles that you can start now and commit to coming back to the others in future, if possible.

Worksheet 2:
In case of emergency . . .

Changing a habit such as comfort eating or bingeing can sometimes be challenging. You may find the following guided exploration really helpful in those moments when you have decided to stop for a minute but are finding it difficult to stay focused and the food is calling insistently.

This worksheet is also available as a guided audio activity which you can download from the Reader's Corner section of our website, dedicated to readers.

Guided exploration

Sit down and take a few deep breaths.

The fact that you have decided to stop eating, maybe just for a few minutes, is an important step forward.

How do you feel? Relieved, anxious, upset?

_____

_____

Think back to when you first realised that you were going to eat in this way, on this occasion . . .

Did you think about it before you even began to eat?

_____

continued

Were you already eating a meal?

_____

Close your eyes for a moment and picture all the details . . .

Where were you?

_____

_____

_____

Who else was there?

_____

_____

_____

What was the atmosphere like?

_____

_____

_____

_____

continued

How were you feeling?

_____

_____

What were you thinking about?

_____

_____

_____

Now picture yourself as you started to overeat or binge . . .

What kind of food did you choose?

_____

_____

_____

How did the food taste? Or didn't you notice?

_____

_____

continued

Were you eating fast or slowly?

_____

_____

What was the food doing for you in that moment?

_____

_____

How were you feeling?

_____

_____

What did you really want?

_____

_____

_____

Put your longing or wish into words or an image . . .

_____

_____

continued

Now feel the relief of having given yourself a few moments to stop.

What do you want to do now?

_____

_____

_____

How are you feeling now? Are you angry, sad, fearful, excited, anxious, lonely?

_____

_____

_____

What would be more nourishing than the food right now?

Do you want to have a good cry?

_____

_____

_____

continued

Would you like to punch a pillow or stamp your feet?

_____

_____

Would you like a hug or a listening ear?

_____

_____

Are you tired and ready for sleep?

_____

_____

Do you want company or would you like to sit alone for a bit?

_____

_____

_____

Whatever you want, whether you can have it or not, acknowledge what it is. If you like putting pen to paper, write about it. If there's someone you can call to talk it through . . . pick up the phone. Decide what you're going to do and when you are ready – do it.

Worksheet 3:
Bring back the joy!

When we are in diet mentality, we are constantly battling with feelings of failure, guilt, inadequacy and frustration. It's easy to forget how wonderful food and eating can be. Remind yourself by considering the following questions and jotting down all the thoughts that come up around food, eating and your body.

Happiness is . . . ?

_____

_____

_____

_____

Pleasure is . . . ?

_____

_____

_____

_____

continued

Fun is . . . ?

_____

_____

_____

_____

_____

_____

Enjoyment is . . . ?

_____

_____

_____

_____

_____

_____

Worksheet 4: Taking stock

Although deep down we know that diets don't work, we want to believe in the magic wands the media and the experts wave at us. The latest miracle solutions are usually backed by 'research'. Do some real research . . . on yourself.

For each diet you've done . . .

Fill in the chart below.

Type of diet	How long did you stay on it?	Did you lose weight?	If yes, how much did you put back on?

Type of diet	How long did you stay on it?	Did you lose weight?	If yes, how much did you put back on?

What is the cost of dieting?

Dieting and being in the diet mentality costs us so much. It wastes time and effort and costs us in terms of our self-esteem and confidence. We also throw away a lot of money on weight-loss schemes.

Do the maths for yourself and find out just how much dieting has cost you. Start by counting the number of years you have spent dieting or trying to lose weight.

TOTAL NUMBER OF YEARS _____

Add up how much money you have spent over the years on dieting, trying to lose weight, staying slim or pummelling your body into the right shape. Our list included things such as:

- diet and recipe books: £____
- expensive ingredients: £____
- membership of WeightWatchers / other slimming clubs: £____
- substitute meals and bars: £____
- gym memberships: £____
- home fitness equipment: £____
- visits to dieticians, nutritionists: £____
- hypnotherapy: £____
- visits to health farms: £____
- hunger suppressants: £____
- herbal integrators: £____
- scales: £____
- calorie charts and counters: £____
- miracle gels and creams: £____
- food conversion charts: £____
- special kitchen equipment: eg steamer / juicer: £____
- Other: £____

TOTAL £_____

Now, take all the money you have spent and divide it by the number of years you have spent on diets – how much have you spent on average each year?

For example, you may have spent £4,000 over a period of 10 years. That's £400 a year.

Whether it works out at £5 or £500 decide what you are going to spend it on over the next 12 months. Whether it's a bunch of flowers or a holiday in the sun it will always be better spent.

I have spent £_____ on average each year

This year I will spend it on _____

_____

_____

_____

_____

_____

_____

_____

_____

_____

_____

_____

_____

Worksheet 5:
What are you waiting for?

There are lots of things that we put off doing, having, or even asking for until we have lost weight. We spend so much time fantasising about a perfect 'thin' life that it's easy to imagine that everything depends on it. We think that life will start when we reach our 'target weight' or when we can get those skinny jeans up past our thighs.

What are you putting off? Make a list below.

1.

2.

3.

4.

5.

Read over your list.

How many of the things on your list have anything to do with weight or body size? We deserve and are worthy of everything, regardless of our weight. Start living now . . . the rest will follow.

Which item on your list will you do this week?

Worksheet 6:
I taste the freedom when . . .

A life Beyond Chocolate is a life of freedom. Virtually all our participants say that the most amazing change in their lives is the sense of freedom . . . free from diets, free from rules and restrictions, free from the limiting belief that the size of our bodies determines the size of our lives.

What does freedom taste like to you?

I taste the freedom when . . .

I taste the freedom when . . .

I taste the freedom when . . .

Further reading

Susan Albers, *Eating Mindfully*, New Herbinger Publications, 2003

Susan Bordo, *Unbearable Weight, Feminism, Western Culture and the Body*, University of California Press, 2003

Paul Campos, *The Obesity Myth: Why America's Obsession with Weight is Hazardous to Your Health*, Gotham Books, 2004

Richard David Carson, *Taming your Gremlin: A surprisingly easy way to get out of your own way*, HarperCollins, 2003 (revised edition)

Pete Cohen, *Habit Busting*, Thorsons, 2002

Nan Kathryn Fuchs, *Overcoming the Legacy of Overeating*, Lowell House, 1997

Judith Duerk, *Circle of Stones*, Inner Ocean Publishing, 2004

Glenn A. Gaesser, *Big Fat Lies: The Truth About Your Weight and Your Health*, Gurze Books, 2002

Jane R. Hirshmann and Carol H. Munter, *Overcoming Overeating: When Women Stop Hating Their Bodies*, Ballantine Books, 1997

Astrid Longhurst, *Body Confidence*, Penguin, 2005

Judith Matz and Ellen Frankel, *Beyond a Shadow of a Diet: The Therapist's Guide to Treating Compulsive Eating*, Brunner-Routlage, 2004

Marilyn Migliore, *The Hunger Within*, Main Street Books, 1998

Rachael Oakes-Ash, *Good Girls Do Swallow*, Mainstream Publishing, 2001

Susie Orbach, *Fat is a Feminist Issue*, Arrow Books 1998

Susie Orbach, *On Eating*, Penguin Books, 2002

Oriah Mountain Dreamer, *The Invitation*, Thorsons, 2000

Carl R. Rogers, *On Becoming a Person*, Constable & Robinson, 2004)

Geneen Roth, *Why Weight? A Guide to Ending Compulsive Eating*, Penguin, 1989

Geneen Roth, *Feeding the Hungry Heart*, Plume, 1993

Geneen Roth, *Appetites*, Plume, 1997

Geneen Roth, *When You Eat at the Refrigerator, Pull Up a Chair*, Hyperion, 1999

Geneen Roth, *Breaking Free from Emotional Eating*, Plume, 2004

Geneen Roth, *When Food is Love*, Plume, 1993

Sark, *Succulent Wild Woman*, Fireside, Simon & Schuster, 1997

Peter N. Stearns, *Fat History: Bodies and Beauty in the Modern West*, New York University Press, 2002

Debra Waterhouse, *Why Women Need Chocolate*, Hyperion, 1996

Naomi Wolf, *The Beauty Myth*, Harper Perennial, 2002

Index

5Rhythms 217–18

all-or-nothing trap 13–27, 154, 193, 211
amino acids 113–14
amphetamines 175
Angel Cards 222
anger 57
Ashford, Claire 169
assertiveness 188–9
audio material 210, 212

babies 38
Balaskas, Kira 218
beaches 128–9
beauty magazines 142
beliefs, personal 182–90, 212, 213
  recognising where they come from
      184–5, 187–8, 195
  updating your 187–8
bile 113
binge eating 2, 53
  between diets 51
  favourite foods for 65
  getting help for 163
  learning to stop 68–71, 74–8, 87–8
  unenjoyable nature of 67
  weekend 3, 17
body
  comparing yours to other women 129,
      131
  defending your 137
  effect of reading beauty magazines on
      your feelings towards 142
  effects of starvation on your 45–6
  flattering your 139
  forming a healthy relationship with
      your 128–43
  hatred of your 2–3, 5, 128–9
  listening to your see tuning in
  naked 136
  owning your 29
  self-talk for your 137, 138
  treats for your 138–9
  water content of the 140

writing a letter to your 137–8
body fat
  creation 112–13
  storage 45
  talking to your 138
body weight
  daily fluctuations 139–41
  see also overweight
boredom, eating and 25, 40, 51
breakfasts 43, 47
  candle-lit 124
Bring Back the Joy (worksheet) 233–4
British Association for Counselling and
      Psychotherapy (BACP) 215–16
British Wheel of Yoga 216–17
bulimia 3

candles 221
carbohydrate cravings 81
changes, making lasting 200
chocolate 64–6, 79–80, 219–20
Chocolate Society, The 220
cholecystokinin 104
chyme 113
clothing 144–50, 204, 213
  dress sizes 148–9
  spring cleans 146, 147–8
confidence 134
cookbooks 124
coping strategies, food as 40, 47–61,
      58–9, 134, 201
counselling 215–16
cravings
  for carbohydrates 81
  satisfying your 76–7, 81
Curtis, Pam 87–8

dance 156, 217–18
Day Chocolate Company 220
desserts 124
detoxes 175
diabetes 201–2
diet diaries 13–16
  see also journals

diets
  all-or-nothing nature of 19, 21
  assessing what type of dieter you are 24
  breaking/slip-ups 65
  costs of 236–8
  difficulties of sticking to 19–20
  effects on your social life 65
  evaluating the effectiveness of 235–6
  first experiences of 2, 4
  hopelessness/failure of 17–21, 26
  mentality of 25, 120
  starvation 45–6, 149
  success/failure yo-yo of 20, 25
  types of 22–3
  and willpower 19–20, 25
  yo-yo 2, 6, 38, 132
digestion 112–14
dinner parties 85, 124
dinners 48, 49
dress sizes 148–9
duodenum 113

Eat Well Nutrition Consultancy 217
eating
  constant 48–9, 95, 122–3
  exactly what you feel like 64–82, 66, 203
  intuitive 177, 180
  night time 48
  quickly
  slowly and mindfully 85–90, 98, 102
    focusing on your food technique 90
    inviting yourself to dinner technique 90–1
    sitting down to eat technique 88–9
    using a plate strategy 85–6, 88, 102, 123
  substitutes to 23–4, 59–60, 211
  whilst doing other things 84–5, 87, 90, 92, 102
  see also binge eating; overeating
eating out 44, 65, 103–4, 123, 187
Eating-Specific Mindfulness Meditation 91
emails, supportive 165–7, 168, 209
emotions
  acknowledging your 50
  identifying your/learning to feel 55–8
  numbing with food 40, 50–5
enjoyment 234
  of food 29, 85–6, 116–26
experimentation, gastronomic 123, 124

experts, being your own 30, 174–81, 182–90, 199–200, 209, 225–40

Fairtrade products 220
fairy cakes 123
families 168
famine/starvation mode 45
fat, dietary 104
  digestion 113
  see also body fat
fear 57
financial matters 217
flavinols 79
flavour of food 125
focusing on food 29, 84–92, 193
food intolerances/allergies 201–2
footcare 221
forbidden foods 64–71
  chocolate 64–6, 79–80
  examples of 73–4
  feeling guilty about eating 120–3
  identifying your 72–4
  learning to eat without bingeing on 68–71, 74–8, 87–8
  learning to enjoy 118–19
  making them abundant 68–9, 75, 77–8, 101, 203–4
  not actually enjoying 67
  secretive/furtive eating of 67–8, 87, 95
  shopping for 77
  worksheet on 211–12
freezing food 112
frequently asked questions 199–205
friends 168
fun 123–4, 234

glycogen stores 140
goals, achievable 193–4
gourmet foods 212
guilt 55, 67, 71, 87–8, 120–3, 134
gurus, being your own 30, 174–81, 182–90, 199–200, 209, 225–40
gyms 156

habits 60
Hall, Jayne 21
Hampshire, Paula P. 169
happiness 57, 131–2, 233
Harris, Kiri 40–1
healthy eating 203
help, asking for 162–72, 195, 213
high-protein diets 17

hunger
    failure to respond to 38–9, 45–6
    psychological effects of 46
    recognising/eating when you are
        hungry 29, 34–46, 47–61,
        98–101, 180, 211
    scale of 41–2
    thinking ahead regarding 44
    waiting too long to eat and 44

I Taste the Freedom When . . .
    (worksheet) 240
In Case of Emergency . . . (worksheet)
    227–32
Internet
    resources 209–14
    shopping for food on the 111
    see also emails
intuitive eaters 177, 180
Irwin, Victoria 71–2, 177–8

jellies 124
Jones, Julie 22
Jonson-Marshall, Caroline 98–9
journals 167–8

Kerslake, Pippa 9–10, 22, 186–7

Layton, Sarah 30–1
Lim, Veronica 217
living in the moment/for today 135, 204,
    239
low-fat foods 102, 104
low-sugar foods 102
lunches 47–8

Macadam, Caro 169
massage, Thai Yoga 218
Mayo Clinic diet 2
McAdam, Caroline 133–4
meditation 91, 216
men 201
menstrual cycle 81, 140
Merrett, Tracey 169
metabolic rate 45
mindless eating 47–61
money management 217
Mouray, Ingrid 166
Munter, Carol 176
muscle, effects of starvation on 45

nakedness 136
neural pathways 60
Newsletter 167

night time eating 48
no, learning to say 188–9
nourishment, alternative sources of
    23–4, 59–60
nutritionists 217

obesity 160
oils, fragrant 221
Orbach, Susie 176
organic food 219
organisations, supportive 215–17
Otis, Carrie 149
overeating 40, 47–61, 134, 201
    ceasing 94–5, 98–9, 200–1
    constant 48–9, 95, 122–3
    and food wastage 106–14
    guided exploration worksheet for
        227–32
    triggers of 58–9
overweight
    physical fitness and 159–60
    secondary benefits of 212

Palazotta, Mauela Alcock 22
pancreas 113
personal development 170
Phull, Surinder 217
physical exercise 30, 117–18, 152–60,
    205, 213
    company for 159
    dance 156, 217–18
    getting started 157–8
    as part of your schedule 159
    yoga 155, 216–17, 218–19
physical fitness 132, 159–60
Pierre Marcolini chocolates 220
Pilates 216
pleasure 119–20, 233
portion sizes 97–8, 101, 103–4
principles of Beyond Chocolate 8–9,
    28–30, 192, 211, 226
protein
    digestion 113–14
    high-protein diets 17
psychotherapy 163, 170, 215–16

Reader's Corner 209, 210–14
reflection 163, 168
retreats 155, 223
Rickards, Sue 217–18
Rococo Chocolates 219
Roth, Geneen 176
running 154

sadness 57
salt intake 140
satiety
  focusing on 102
  recognising 29, 37, 41, 68, 94–105,
    106–14, 180, 212
  and snacking 61
scales 139–41
secretive/furtive eating 67–8, 87, 95,
  163
self-appreciation 194
self-awareness 195
self-confidence 134
self-hatred 2–3, 5, 128–9
self-talk 137, 138
serotonin 81
Seventypercent.com 219–20
shopping for food
  honest 111–12
  on the Internet 111
  to avoid wastage 111–12
slimming pills 175
snacking
  day-long 48–9, 122–3
  when not hungry 61
social lives, effects of dieting on 65
Spectrum 215
spring cleans, for your wardrobe 146,
  147–8
starting Beyond Chocolate 191–8
starvation diets 45–6, 149
starvation mode 45
Stavely-Hill, Lexi 21
Stevens, Kay 122–3
support 30, 162–72
  from families and friends 168
  organisations for 215–17
  relying on food for 40, 134
  through emails 165–7, 168, 209

Taking Stock (worksheet) 235–8
tasting sessions, guided 212
tea 221–2
tea parties 123
Thai Yoga Massage 218
thinness
  and happiness 131–2
  and physical fitness 159–60
  society's privileging of 131
treats, for your body 138–9

triggers, of overeating 58–9
Triyoga 216
tuning in 28–31, 37, 39, 41–3, 202
  assessing your hunger levels 37, 39,
    41–3, 52
  identifying what you really fancy to
    eat 78–9
  identifying your emotions 56–8
  and physical exercise 158
  recognising satiety 96–8
  reminders for 42–3
  taking the time for 204–5

vanity sizing 149
vomiting, to control weight 2

walking 160
wasting food 106–14
water content of the body 140
weight control methods 23–4, 59–60,
  211
  see also diets
weight loss, success 202–3
WeightWatchers 2, 4, 89
What Are You Waiting For? (worksheet)
  239
Williams, Eileen 169
Williams, Gareth 218–19
willpower 19–20, 25, 65, 200–1
Wilson, Cathie 156, 196–7
Wolf, Naomi 176
Woman Within 216
women, pressures of 165
worksheets 209–10, 211–12, 213,
  225–40
  Bring Back the Joy 233–4
  I Taste the Freedom When . . . 240
  In Case of Emergency . . . 227–32
  Taking Stock 235–8
  What Are You Waiting For? 239
  Your Expert Opinion 225–6
workshops 169–70, 223–4
written exercises 209–10
  describing your relationship with food
    178–9
  journals 167–8

yo-yo dieting 2, 6, 38, 132
yoga 155, 216–17, 218–19
Your Expert Opinion (worksheet) 225–6